Ahmad
Esthetic Clinical Case Studies

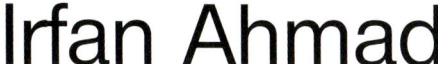

Irfan Ahmad

Esthetic Clinical Case Studies: Dilemmas and Solutions

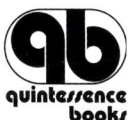

Quintessence Publishing Co, Ltd
London, Berlin, Chicago, Tokyo, Barcelona, Beijing, Istanbul, Milan,
Moscow, Mumbai, Paris, Prague, São Paulo, and Warsaw

A book for Zayan

British Library Cataloguing in Publication Data
Esthetic Clinical Case Studies: Dilemmas and Solutions
   1. Dentistry – Aesthetic aspects
   I. Title
   617.6
   ISBN-13: 978-1-85097-172-6

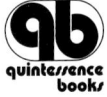

© 2009 Quintessence Publishing Co, Ltd

Quintessence Publishing Co, Ltd
Grafton Road
New Malden
Surrey KT3 3AB
United Kingdom
www.quintpub.co.uk

All rights reserved. This book or any part thereof may not be reproduced, stored in a retrieval system, or transmitted in any form or by any means, electronic, mechanical, photocopying, or otherwise, without prior written permission of the publisher.

Cover image by Irfan Ahmad
ISBN-13: 978-1-85097-172-6
Printed in Germany

Preface

There are three aspects to learning: theoretical, procedural, and performance. Each one is necessary for learning a given task. The objective of this book is to concentrate on performance. Performance is doing – it is clinical practice. It is the part of the learning process that builds experience, through learning from mistakes and, most importantly, self-deprecation – with the view that improvement is infinite, never finite, no matter how good the performance. It is worth remembering that perfection is a journey, not a destination.

This book works on two levels. First, it can be used in conjunction with other textbooks, dealing with theoretical and procedural aspects, and second, it can be read as a standalone text to aid critical thinking and treatment planning, which are essential for performance. For this reason, references are omitted, and the reader should consult dental literature or Internet search engines for more information on the theory or technique that is under discussion.

An effective method for teaching performance is to use case studies depicting clinical challenges and demonstrating how dilemmas can be transformed into solutions. Therefore, this book is mainly pictorial, with sparse text. The text serves to guide the reader to salient items of the planning process or clinical practice. The premise of the book is to present a variety of anterior dental esthetic anomalies, and then propose options (which are not exhaustive) for solving each of these dilemmas. After discussing the "pros and cons" of each option, one is chosen to restore health, function, and esthetics.

For any given disorder, there is often more than one option for treatment, but the key element is to adopt a systematic, evidence-based approach to treatment planning (outlined in Chapter 1). The chapters in this book cover a wide range of prosthodontic modalities, including porcelain laminate veneers, full-coverage crowns, fixed partial dentures, and dental implants. The option chosen for treating a specific anomaly is neither right nor wrong, but is one method for achieving the desired outcome. It is hoped that presenting different options, and the reasons for pursuing a particular option, will stimulate discussion and help with the thought process during this crucial and vital stage of any therapy. No doubt some will agree with the chosen options, while others will beg to differ. If this is the case, the book will have accomplished its task.

The layout of the book is as follows. Chapter 1 describes the evidence-based treatment approach for methodical treatment planning. The remaining chapters each discuss a case study with one or more dental esthetic dilemmas. These chapters have an identical format.

1. Pre- and postoperative status
2. Dental history
3. Preoperative status
4. Treatment options
5. Scientific credence for treatment
6. Clinical erudition and feasibility
7. Patient needs and wants (and reasons for choosing a particular option)
8. Treatment sequence (detailing clinical and laboratory sequences for the chosen option)
9. Discussion.

Items 5, 6, and 7 form the evidence-based treatment planning approach discussed in Chapter 1.

Adopting this consistent format ensures uniformity in the treatment planning process, allowing the reader to apply these steps for their own patients. Although the cases shown are all related to anterior dental esthetics, this approach is useful for arriving at eventual solutions for all types of clinical dilemma.

The making of this book has been possible with the participation, and kind permission, of the featured patients. Many of the pictures depicting various clinical stages are beyond those necessary for treatment, and I am thankful to my patients for their endurance and for giving up their valuable time. Without this altruistic co-operation, the book would not have come to fruition. I am also thankful to Dr Alan Sidi for carrying out some of the surgical procedures, and to all the dental technicians who have produced stunning ceramics for the definitive restorations. In addition, my gratitude goes to the Quintessence "production machinery" for translating my thoughts into reality, and especially Mr Haase for accepting this project for publication.

Irfan Ahmad

Contents

Chapter 1
Evidence-based Treatment Planning   1

Chapter 2
Replacing Congenitally Missing Maxillary
Canines and Lateral Incisors   9

Chapter 3
Restoring Structural Integrity and Esthetics
Following Tooth Wear   21

Chapter 4
Declining Fortunes of Two Maxillary Incisors   39

Chapter 5
Traumatic Loss of Maxillary Central Incisors   55

Chapter 6
Vicissitudes of Two Maxillary Incisors
Over 21 Years   63

Chapter 7
Restitution of Anterior Dental Esthetics with a
Variety of Restorations   95

Chapter 8
A Single Maxillary Central Incisor with
a Hopeless Prognosis   109

Evidence-based Treatment Planning

1 Evidence-based Treatment Planning

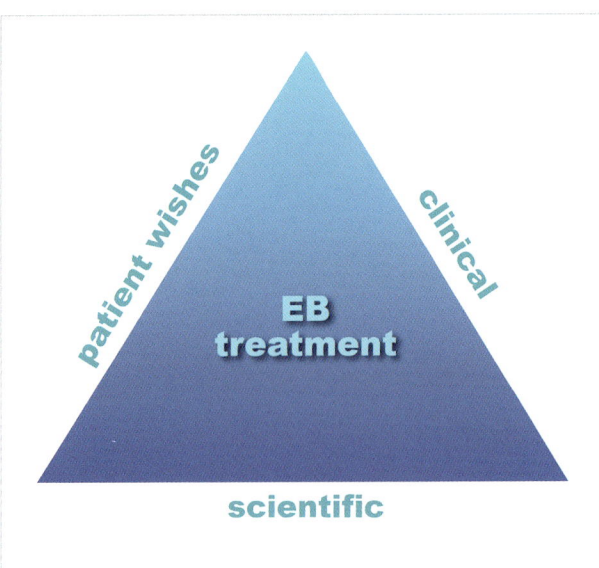

Fig 1-1 Equilateral triangle representing an evidence-based (EB) treatment plan where all three factors – clinical, scientific, and patient wishes – are equally represented.

Throughout their lives in practice, most practitioners are confronted with clinical dilemmas and the need to search for therapeutic solutions. In each case, clinical decisions impact on the treatment delivered, affecting oral health and the longevity of the dentition. The chosen treatment option may be a success or result in failure, and the outcome is primarily determined at the planning stage. Therefore, pitfalls should be foreseen and strategically circumvented by careful planning. But are guidelines available to help practitioners to avoid catastrophes? In absolute terms, and with the best intentions in the world, there are no guarantees of predicting and ensuring a successful outcome. However, there are steps that can be taken to maximize success and minimize failure.

One such step is to adopt the fundamental ethos of treatment planning – that is, a systematic approach. The first stage of planning is gathering information, including medical and dental histories, examinations, and requisite tests and investigations. After collating this information, a diagnosis is reached, which determines options for alleviating symptoms and resolving ailments.

Although information gathering and diagnosis are reasonably objective protocols, the ensuing treatment options can be, and often are, tainted by subjectivity. Subjectivity per se is not detrimental, but a systematic approach must be adopted and a rationale offered for arriving at a specific proposal or set of proposals.

A systematic, evidence-based (EB) approach to treatment planning can be imagined as an equilateral triangle, with the sides representing the three key factors: scientific rationale, clinical erudition and feasibility, and patient needs and wants (Fig 1-1). Ideally, all three factors should be represented in equal proportions, and their combination results in a bespoke treatment plan tailored to a given clinical predicament. In reality, however, one factor will predominate, while the others are present in lesser proportions. For example, if an operator

1 Evidence-based Treatment Planning

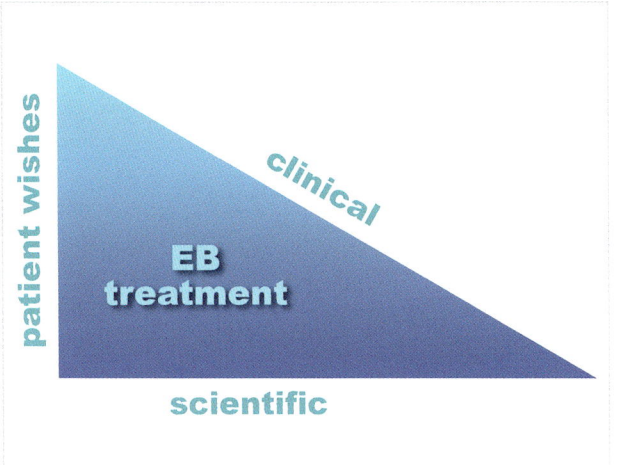

Fig 1-2 Unequal triangle representing an evidence-based (EB) treatment plan that has a bias in favor of the clinician.

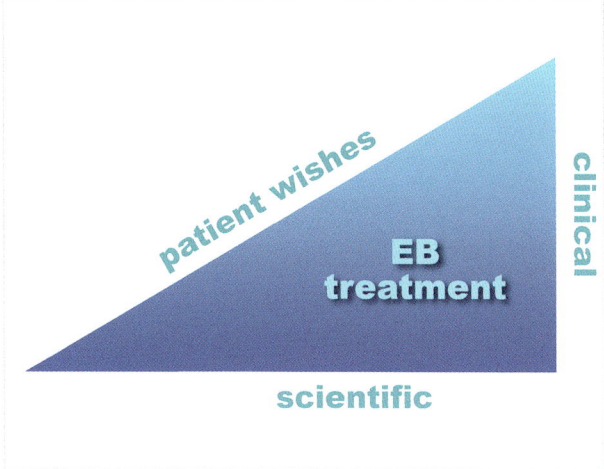

Fig 1-3 Unequal triangle representing an evidence-based (EB) treatment plan that has a bias in favor of patient wishes.

(clinical) has a penchant for a particular treatment, the triangle will not be equilateral but will show a bias in favor of the clinician (Fig 1-2). Conversely, if patient wishes predominate, the patient factor prejudices a particular course of treatment (Fig 1-3).

Of course each of the three factors itself covers a range of variables, but this formula provides the basis for a reliable, systematic approach. A haphazard or slapdash approach will usually yield unpredictable outcomes.

Scientific Rationale

The first part of EB treatment planning is to establish the scientific basis for the proposed treatment options. The questions to ask about the proposed treatment are:
- Does it have scientific credence?
- Does it fulfill the health, function, and esthetics triad?
- What is the success or survival rate?
- Is it ethical?

Scientific Credence

The main question here is which, out of all the options available to treat an anomaly, are scientifically sound? For example, to improve the esthetics of a heavily restored, discolored maxillary central incisor, the following could be considered:
- bleaching, with or without direct composite fillings
- porcelain laminate veneer
- all-ceramic crown
- metal-ceramic crown

- extraction and removable partial denture
- extraction and fixed partial denture
- extraction and implant.

The scientific rationale for each option should be justified depending on the clinical findings and diagnosis of the discoloration. If the tooth is vital and the discoloration is caused by stained and/or defective composite restorations, then the most suitable option would be replacement fillings. Alternatively, if the discoloration is intrinsic owing to loss of vitality and the tooth is root filled, the most appropriate and least invasive option would be bleaching in conjunction with new fillings. However, if the root filling is deficient (with apical radiolucency), bleaching and new fillings would be contraindicated. In these circumstances, the most appropriate action would be a replacement root filling. But what if there is a history of previously failed root fillings and apicectomies? If this is the case, attempting another root filling would be futile and may even be counterproductive. Extraction and a prosthesis to close the space would perhaps yield a better prognosis.

This example demonstrates two crucial aspects to consider before pursuing a course of treatment. First, a definitive diagnosis is essential, and second, the therapeutic modality must be supported by recent research.

Health, Function and Esthetics

The next item to consider under the scientific category is whether or not the treatment options fulfill the health, function, and esthetics triad. The aims of any treatment should follow a hierarchical sequence. The paramount priority is health: health of the periodontium and tooth. This is followed by function: occlusion and phonetics. It is only after the latter is achieved that esthetics can be contemplated. If this sequence is ignored, the treatment is doomed to failure. For example, providing a beautiful all-ceramic crown may fulfill the esthetic aims, but if the surrounding periodontium is unhealthy, disaster is imminent. Similarly, fitting an all-ceramic crown for a bruxist or for someone with a steep anterior guidance is also ill fated.

Survival Rates

Most patients desiring esthetic improvement will also wish to know the survival rate of what is being proposed. While it is impossible to predict with certainty the longevity of a particular restoration, and many in-vitro trials are not representative of a clinical environment, scientific data can nevertheless be used as a guide for average survival or success rates. For example, an all-ceramic crown on an incisor has a higher survival rate than a similar crown on a molar. If esthetics is a priority, then an all-ceramic unit is the ideal choice, but if longevity is the overriding concern, a metal-ceramic unit may be more appropriate. The key issue is to inform the patient before starting treatment, thereby avoiding ambiguity or blame in the event of an unfavorable outcome.

Ethics

The last item to consider is ethics. Ethics consists of four main principles:
- non-malfeasance – "doing no harm" (the Hippocratic principle); for example, perhaps not fulfilling patients' wishes but at least not harming them
- beneficence – ensuring the well-being of patients
- autonomy – veracity in clinician–patient relationships
- justice – fairness and impartiality.

To be strictly ethical, adherence to all four of the above principles is a prerequisite. If one or more is not observed, ethics are compromised. In reality, however, one or more principles prevail at the expense of the others. Compromises are usually made because of differences of opinion between the patient and the clinician, with one party dictating and the other accepting.

Esthetic dentistry often presents a challenge for ethics because patients' wishes may conflict with clinical necessity. This is increasingly becoming a contentious issue. The best advice is to adhere to dental ethics, which may mean refusing treatment that is construed as a want rather than a need. At times, saying "no" at the outset is a positive action and will avoid possible future argument or litigation.

Clinical Erudition and Feasibility

The second part of EB treatment is clinical erudition and feasibility. The questions to ask are:
- Does the clinician and/or ceramist have the knowledge?
- Does the clinician and/or ceramist have the skill?
- Does the clinician and/or ceramist have the experience?

Knowledge

Knowledge is learned, not inherently possessed. Knowledge is the first step in learning about a technique or procedure. Knowledge is also essential for keeping abreast of the latest scientific advances and current thinking. Depending on aptitude and schedule, a clinician can gain knowledge by reading books, watching videos, attending symposia or participating in hands-on courses. Besides fulfilling the mandatory hourly requirements for professional registration or a license to practice, learning is probably the best way to help patients. It allows clinicians to offer treatment options based on current research, superseding outdated thinking and methodologies.

Skill

There are two theories about talent (or skill). The first is that talent is inborn, and the second is that it is learned. The former theory stipulates that an individual has an innate talent for carrying out a specific task. Painters, sculptors, writers, singers and surgeons are often said to be talented in this way. The alternate theory is characterized by the analogy of a dog with a bone. A dog perseveres with biting the hard cortex of the bone until it is rewarded with the inner soft bone marrow. Effectively, the dog possesses no talent but eventually accomplishes the task through intrepidness and endurance. Whichever theory one subscribes to – innate talent or success through perseverance – is irrelevant. The salient point is that talent (skill) is necessary to perform a given task.

Knowledge is invaluable for teaching a skill, but knowledge alone is insufficient for performing a procedure. A skill is perfected with practice, and a major advantage of hands-on courses is that knowledge is practically applied for specific clinical techniques.

Clinical self-awareness is essential, and if a clinician feels that he or she cannot deliver a chosen course of treatment, referral is the best option. Referral at this early stage is prudent and instills confidence in the patient. It avoids facing a cul-de-sac later or having no choice but to refer when things go wrong.

In some parts of the world, however, specialist referral is impractical. In these situations, one could consider a simpler and more manageable treatment, which might not be ideal but would be practical given the particular circumstances. Treatment that seems invasive and destructive in one part of the world might be the only option for achieving health in another location. It is important to realize, and to reserve judgment, that one cannot transpose the values of one country (or one dental practice) into another without first knowing the facts and circumstances of that particular locality or practice.

Experience

The last clinical aspect to consider is experience. Experience is the result of making mistakes. No mistakes, no experience! Once the necessary knowledge and skills for a given procedure or specialty are acquired, experience will ensure that it is delivered predictably and that pitfalls are avoided.

Experience develops with time and cannot be rushed; it is the perpetual distillation of theory and application over years of practice. The key factor to emphasize is that experience is the result of repetition: the more a procedure is performed, the greater the experience.

Finally, experience allows the feasibility of a treatment option to be determined. Even if a therapy is scientifically sound and the clinician and ceramist have the necessary skills, the feasibility (and eventual outcome) of a procedure can only be assessed if the operators have the necessary experience to make a sound judgment.

Patient Needs and Wants

The last part of EB treatment is to consider patient needs and wants. The questions to ask are:
- Can the patient afford the treatment?
- Can the patient endure the treatment?
- Does the patient want the treatment?

Cost of Treatment

Cost can often be the deciding factor for a patient to proceed with or decline a course of treatment. For some patients, cost is irrelevant and plays little or no part during the decision-making process. For others, cost is paramount, and if excessive may result in refusal of treatment. However, cost need not be a deciding factor for achieving dental health. As previously mentioned, there is usually more than one option for achieving health, and although the cheapest option may not be the state-of-the-art in dental care, it can nevertheless achieve dental health for many who would otherwise reject therapy. Furthermore, offering a less-expensive option is better than offering no options and losing a patient. In addition, if the patient's finances improve in the future, he or she will be more likely to attend the same practice for more sophisticated treatment.

Duration of Treatment

It is often tempting to offer patients the best available treatment. But the best option may also be the most protracted, and it is necessary to consider whether the patient is capable of enduring a lengthy, drawn-out treatment plan. If the patient is elderly, or medically or physically impaired, compliance with prolonged treatment is likely to be poor. Once again, a simpler option may achieve health and satisfy the patient's present dental needs, but with functional and/or esthetic compromises.

Patient wants

Responses from patients to recommended treatment plans may include reticence or rejection. While clinicians strive to offer the latest treatment options, there are occasions when the patient is not interested in elaborate or involved therapies. Besides financial constraints, the patient may not cherish the thought of dental treatment, may harbor dental phobias, or not prioritize dental health. For these reasons, the patient may genuinely not wish to have the most esthetically available crown, and may prefer to accept a compromise.

At the other extreme, patients may dictate a specific treatment plan involving extensive and expensive protocols. For example, whitening teeth from an A3 to A1 shade may be possible with bleaching, but the patient may reject this proposal and insist on having porcelain laminate veneers to achieve the same objective. In these situations, clinicians are in a quandary: should they bow to patient pressure or should they stick to scientific principles? The answer lies in each clinician's judgment of whether the patient's requests can be delivered without compromising the ethical standards of the profession.

Conclusion

From the above discussion, it is obvious that treatment planning is fraught with subjectivity. Many factors influence the decisions of both practitioners and patients. The final treatment plan is a combination of these unique differences, which are often not reproducible in another practice with another clinician. However, a good starting point is to use a systematic EB model; a disorganized approach will increase the likelihood of erratic outcomes.

Replacing Congenitally Missing Maxillary Canines and Lateral Incisors

2

Diagnostic waxup and surgical stent by Gérald Ubassy, Avignon, France
Ceramics by Stephen Chu and Adam Mieleszko, NYU, New York, USA

Pre- and Postoperative Status

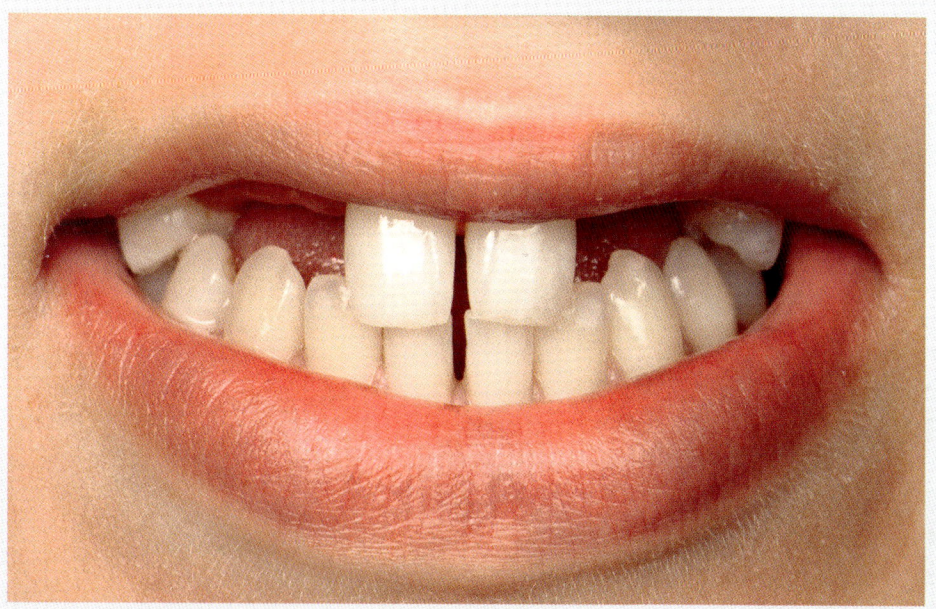

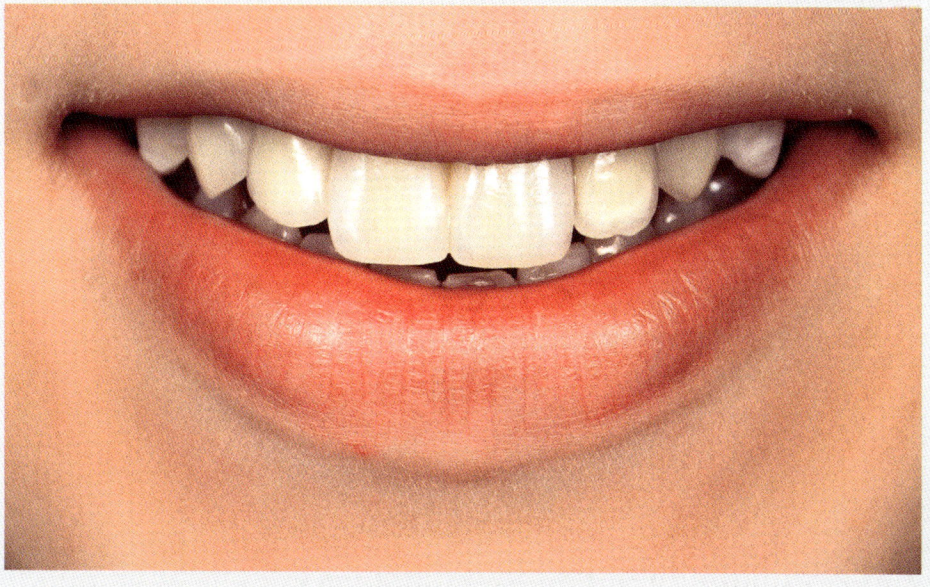

2 Replacing Congenitally Missing Maxillary Canines and Lateral Incisors

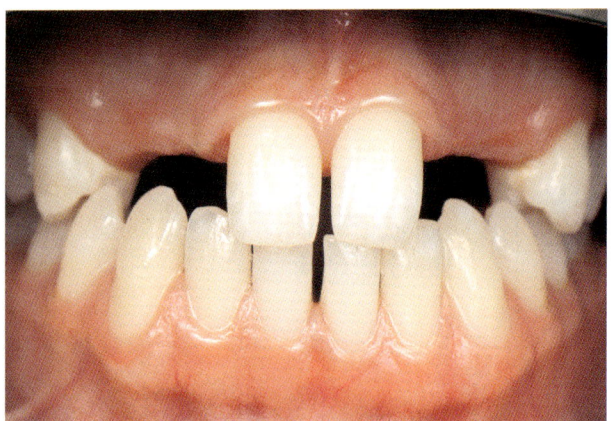

Fig 2-1 Preoperative anterior view.

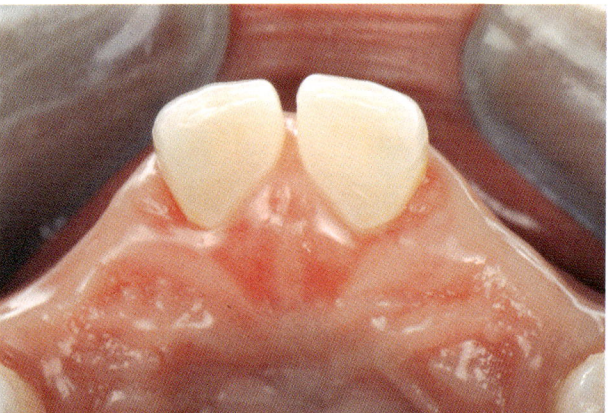

Fig 2-2 Preoperative incisal view.

Dental History

A young woman, 19 years of age, wished to improve her anterior dental esthetic predicament. She presented with congenitally missing maxillary canines and lateral incisors (Figs 2-1 and 2-2) and had worn a removable acrylic-resin partial denture since the age of 12 years, when she became socially aware. In addition, she disliked the narrow maxillary central incisors, which lacked dominance and detracted from a pleasing smile.

Preoperative Status

Intraoral examination revealed median maxillary and mandibular diastemata, with a reduced mesial–distal width of the central incisors (small width to length ratio). The atrophic alveolar ridge at the sites of the missing teeth was deficient, with both a horizontal and vertical defect.

Treatment Options

1. A removable acrylic-resin partial denture, and mesial resin-composite fillings for the central incisors to close the diastema and improve morphology (increasing the width to length ratio) (Fig 2-3).
2. Two four-unit fixed partial dentures (FPDs), using the first premolars and central incisors as abutments (Fig 2-4).
3. Four implant-supported crowns at the lateral incisor and canine sites, and mesial resin-composite fillings or two porcelain laminate veneers (PLVs) for the central incisors (Fig 2-5).
4. Two implants at the canine sites, with two three-unit FPDs using the implants and central incisors as abutments (Fig 2-6).
5. Two implants at the canine sites with two two-unit implant-supported cantilever bridges, and resin-composite fillings or two PLVs for the central incisors (Fig 2-7).

2 Replacing Congenitally Missing Maxillary Canines and Lateral Incisors

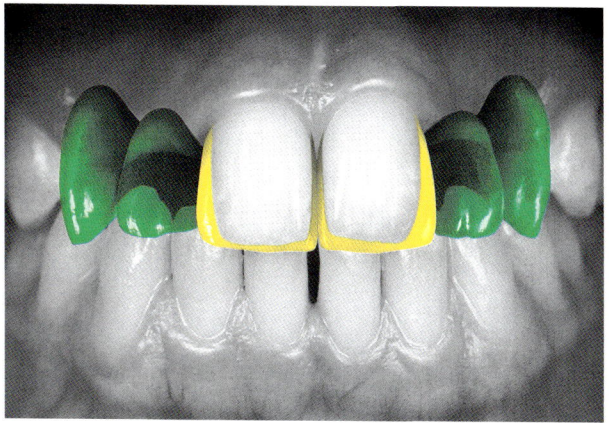

Fig 2-3 Option 1: an acrylic-resin removable partial denture (green) and mesial resin-composite fillings (yellow).

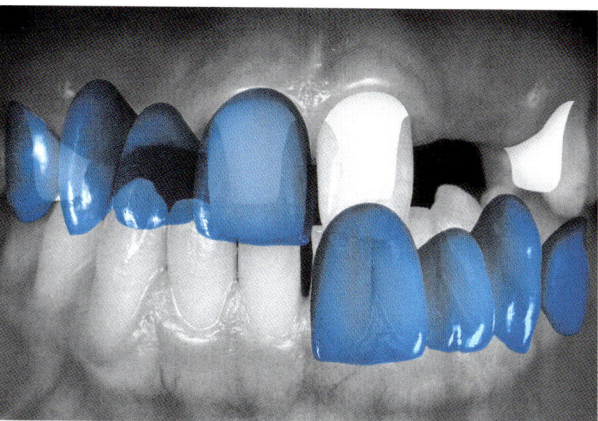

Fig 2-4 Option 2: two four-unit FPDs (blue), using the first premolars and central incisors as abutments.

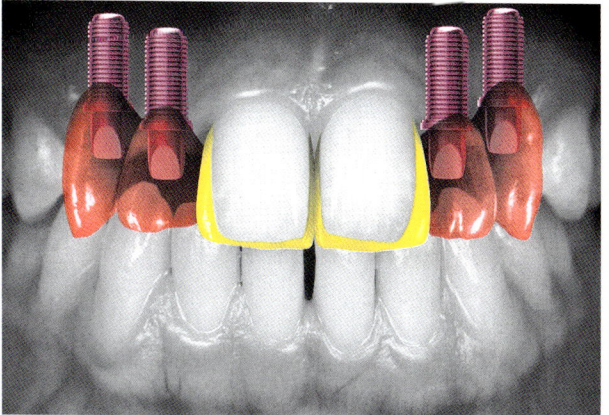

Fig 2-5 Option 3: four implant-supported crowns (red), and mesial resin-composite fillings or two PLVs for the central incisors (yellow).

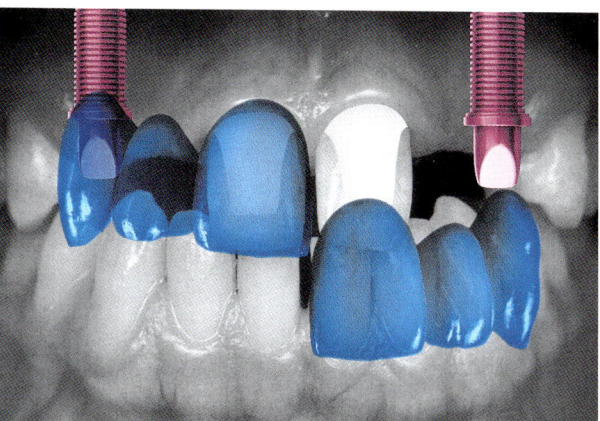

Fig 2-6 Option 4: two implants at canine sites, with two three-unit FPDs (blue) using the implants and central incisors as abutments.

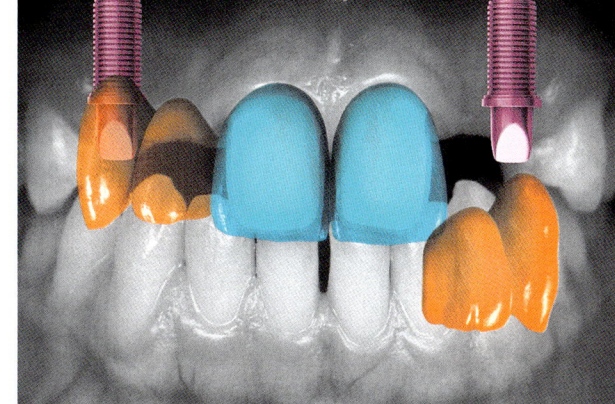

Fig 2-7 Option 5: two implants at the canine sites with two two-unit implant-supported cantilever bridges (orange), and resin-composite fillings or two PLVs for the central incisors (turquoise).

11

Scientific Credence for Treatment Options

A partial denture is prone to dislodgement, and in a young patient can be socially embarrassing. The advantage of direct resin-composite fillings is minimal invasion – little or no tooth preparation is required. However, resin composite is likely to wear and stain, requiring periodic maintenance and polishing. Tooth preparation of four vital, healthy teeth for FPDs is highly destructive, and may result in possible future endodontic complications.

Considering the narrow alveolar ridge, augmentation (soft and hard tissue) is a prerequisite for placing implants. The esthetic outcome is generally better when fewer implants are used to restore missing teeth. Hence, placing four implants can be an esthetic compromise. Furthermore, depending on the diameter of the fixtures, it is essential to ensure a mesial–distal distance of 2.5 mm between teeth and implants and a space of 3 mm between implants. Consequently, space limitations could be a contraindication for placing four implants. Compared with direct composite fillings, PLVs require more aggressive tooth preparation, but they yield better long-term esthetics, assuming that adequate enamel is retained to maintain tooth rigidity and for bonding with a resin luting agent.

Linking natural teeth to implants using an FPD has caused some concerns, and the dental literature has reported instances of intrusion and/or disuse atrophy. However, research and clinical findings at this time are inconclusive regarding the long-term effects of using this modality.

Placing fewer implants is obviously less traumatic and costly as there is less surgery. In addition, sculpting the pontic sites with ovate-shaped provisional restorations simulates natural emergence profiles, thereby enhancing esthetics. But cantilever bridges have a propensity for unwanted rotation, and if occlusion is not meticulously addressed, dislodgement is a frequent occurrence. In this instance, the guiding canine teeth are being replaced with implants, and group function using the premolars rather than canine guidance may be prudent during lateral excursion. The advantage of using cantilever bridges is that linking natural teeth with implants is obviated.

Clinical Erudition and Feasibility

The first two options – a removable partial denture or a FPD – are within the remit of a general practitioner. The implant options require surgical training and experience, which may necessitate referral or a second opinion.

Patient Needs and Wants

If finances were a concern, the first option would be the most appropriate. However, the patient had no financial constraints, and since she had worn and disliked a removable denture for the previous 7 years, her wishes were to seek a fixed prosthodontic solution. With four teeth already missing, the patient was

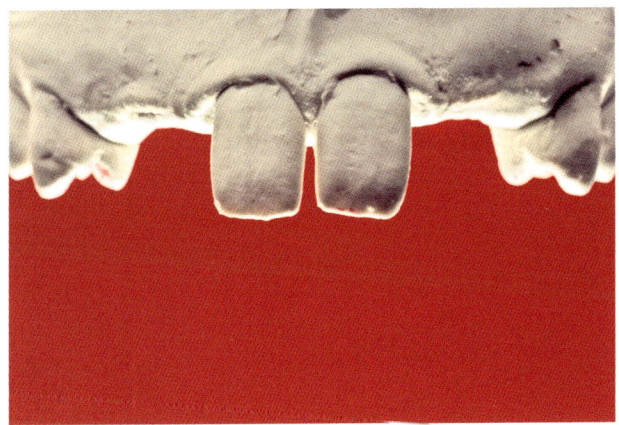

Fig 2-8 Preoperative plaster cast: anterior view.

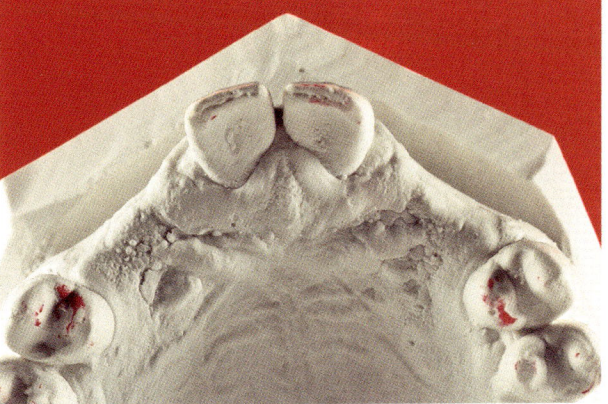

Fig 2-9 Preoperative plaster cast: incisal view.

reluctant to prepare another four healthy teeth, which could result in endodontic problems, or even future extractions. Therefore, her choice was the implant route. After explaining the scientific rationale for using fewer implants and not linking teeth with implants, she veered to being cautious by accepting option 5, with knowledge of the drawbacks of cantilever bridges (rotation and dislodgement) and PLVs (tooth reduction).

Treatment Sequence

The preoperative articulated casts (Figs 2-8 and 2-9) revealed group function on the premolars (red articulation-paper marks). Since the canines were being replaced with implant-supported prostheses, it was essential to ensure that group function on the premolars was maintained to avoid undue stress on the fixtures and eventual cantilever bridges.

A diagnostic waxup allowed assessment and feasibility of the proposed treatment plan, as well as appraisal of the morphology, alignment, and space availability of the maxillary anterior sextant. Use of tooth-colored wax facilitates communication with patients and helps to gauge the envisaged esthetic outcome (Figs 2-10 and 2-11). The waxup also serves as a template for a transitional acrylic-resin partial denture, surgical stent and morphology of the definitive prostheses.

To fabricate the transitional partial denture, the preoperative plaster cast was trimmed at the canine and lateral sites to simulate ovate pontics (Fig 2-12). The acrylic-resin teeth were shaped to fit the ovate sites for sculpting the overlying soft tissues during the osseointegration phase (Fig 2-13).

The stent from the waxup was used as a guide for fixture placement at the canine sites (Figs 2-14 and 2-15).

Owing to the maxillary horizontal and vertical ridge defect, a two-stage surgical procedure was planned. Using the stent, two Branemark Mk III, 3.75 mm RP (Nobel Biocare, Sweden) fixtures were placed concurrent with bone grafting using Bio-Oss (Geistlich, Switzerland) and connective tissue grafts from the

2 Replacing Congenitally Missing Maxillary Canines and Lateral Incisors

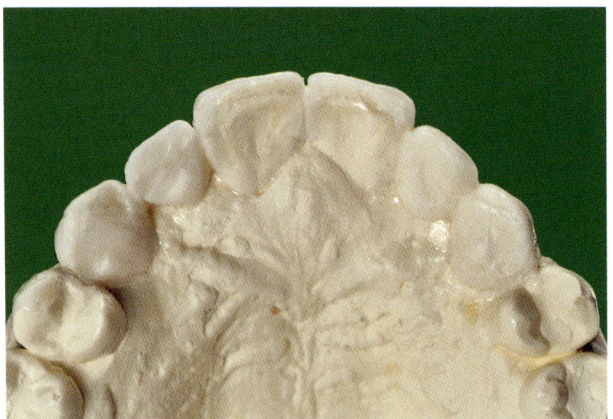

Fig 2-10 Diagnostic waxup: incisal view.

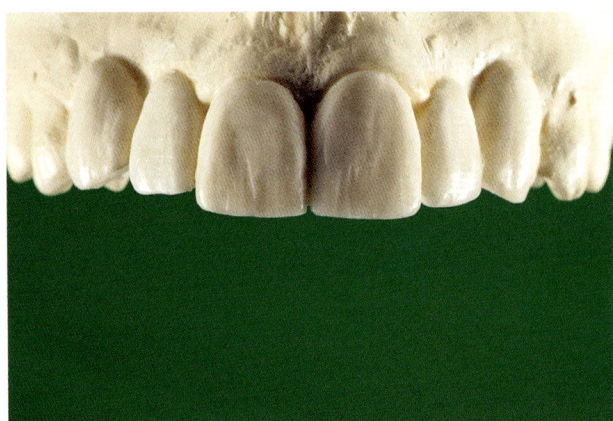

Fig 2-11 Diagnostic waxup: anterior view.

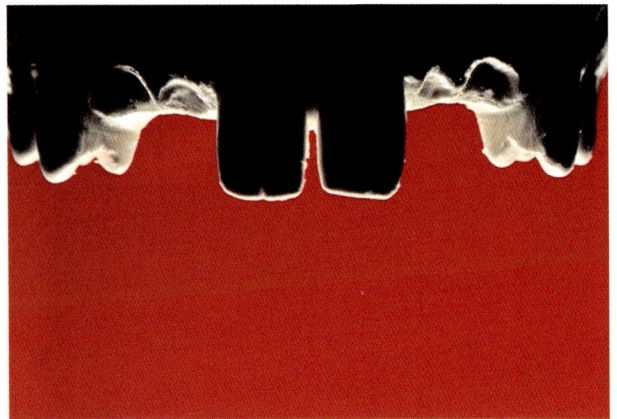

Fig 2-12 Preoperative plaster cast with trimmed ovate pontics at lateral incisor and canine sites.

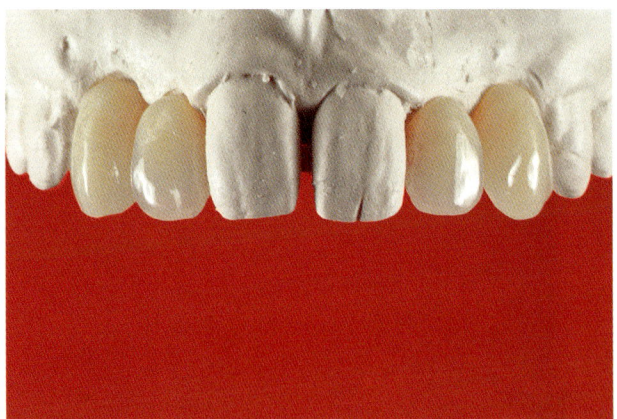

Fig 2-13 Transitional acrylic-resin partial denture.

palate (Figs 2-16 and 2-17). The transitional denture was adjusted and fitted after the surgery.

At 3 months, the surgical sites were healing without incidence and the tissues were being sculptured by the denture (Figs 2-18 and 2-19). At 6 months, soft tissue sculpturing at the canine and lateral sites was clearly evident (Figs 2-20 and 2-21). Although the gingival scallop was well defined, the tissue was thin and the patient at this stage was offered further grafting from the palate. However, the patient declined additional grafting and accepted the compromise of possible 'shine through' of a titanium implant abutment. However, using a ceramic abutment with superior light transmission can mitigate the unwanted cervical shadowing. Furthermore, the lip line is low, which would probably conceal the cervical areas of the cantilever bridges.

2 Replacing Congenitally Missing Maxillary Canines and Lateral Incisors

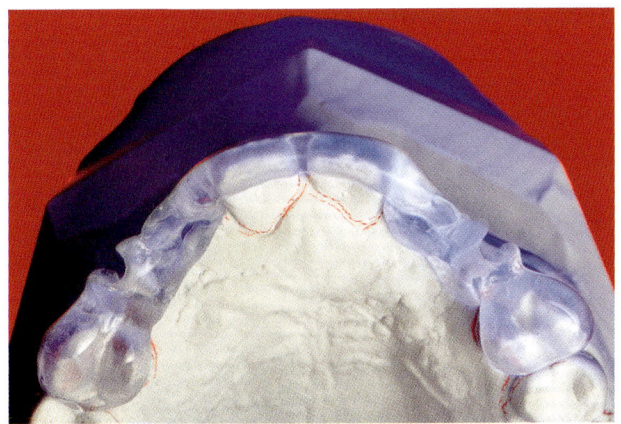

Fig 2-14 Surgical stent with drill guides at canine sites: incisal view.

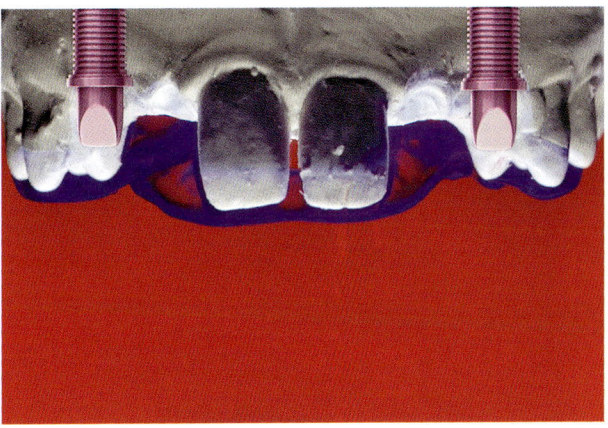

Fig 2-15 Surgical stent with drill guides at canine sites and proposed implant location: anterior view.

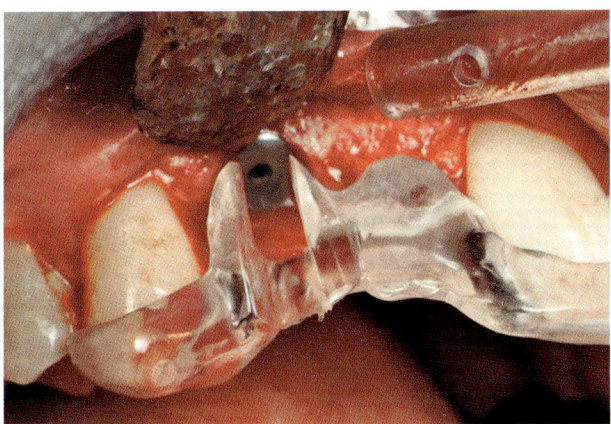

Fig 2-16 Surgical stent in situ for guiding implant fixture placement at right canine site.

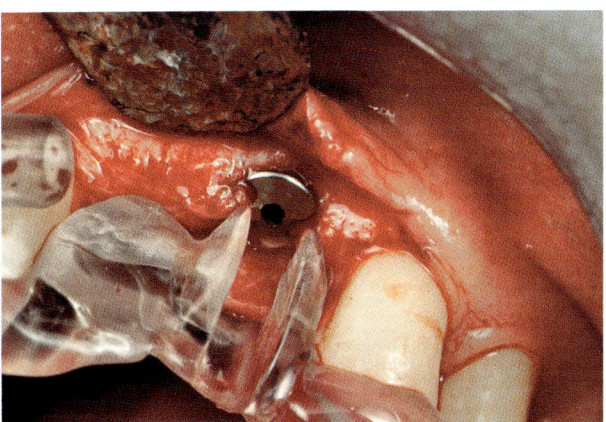

Fig 2-17 Surgical stent in situ for guiding implant fixture placement at left canine site.

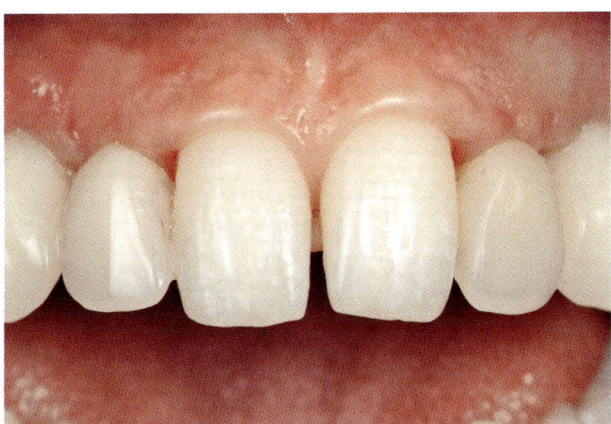

Fig 2-18 Acrylic-resin partial denture in situ at 3 months.

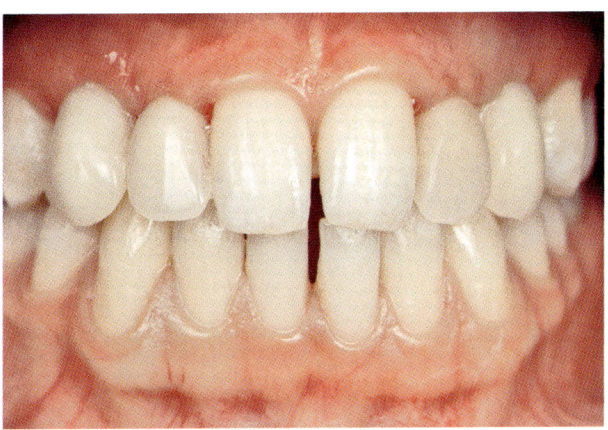

Fig 2-19 Acrylic-resin partial denture in situ at 3 months.

2 Replacing Congenitally Missing Maxillary Canines and Lateral Incisors

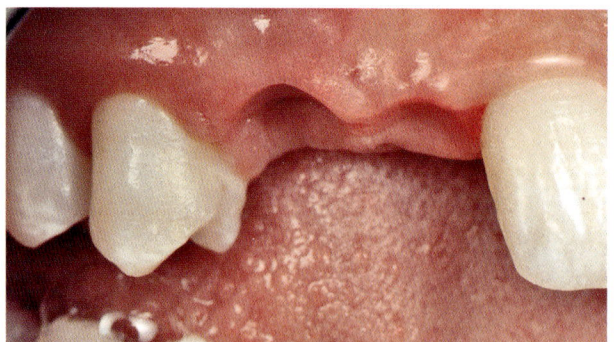

Fig 2-20 Sculptured soft tissues at the right lateral incisor and canine sites following 6 months of wearing the acrylic-resin partial denture.

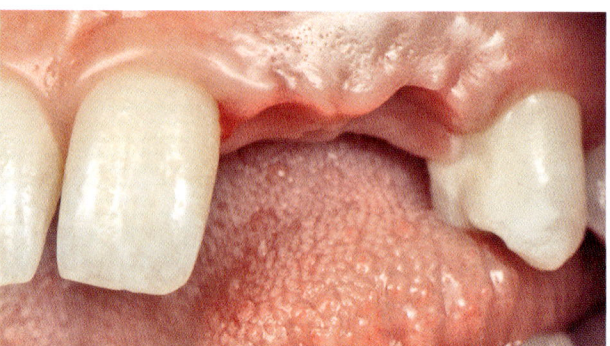

Fig 2-21 Sculptured soft tissues at the left lateral incisor and canine sites following 6 months of wearing the acrylic-resin partial denture.

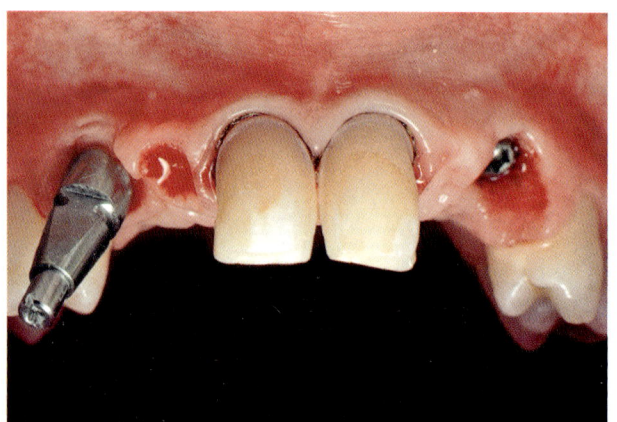

Fig 2-22 PLV tooth preparations for central incisors and an impression coping in situ on right implant fixture.

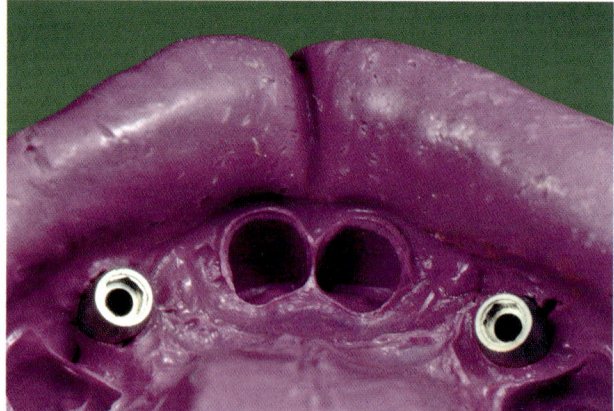

Fig 2-23 Maxillary impression with embedded copings recording the sculpted tissues at the lateral incisor and canine sites and PLV preparations on the central incisors.

The maxillary central incisors were prepared for PLVs, and an impression was made using impression copings on the fixtures. Notice the severe angulations of the fixtures, necessitating custom-made abutments (Figs 2-22 and 2-23). Soft-tissue models were poured, and abutments fabricated of cast gold with circumferential alumina porcelain shoulders (Figs 2-24 and 2-25).

An important point about implant abutments is that the transmucosal part should be either titanium or alumina, or possibly zirconia. The reason is that these three materials encourage epithelial and connective attachment, forming a soft tissue cuff to guard against bacterial invasion or mechanical insult. Materials such as cast metals or silica-based ceramics should not contact the transmucosal tissue cuff as they do not allow epithelial or connective tissue attachments. Also, the abutment shape at the cervical region should be flat or

2 Replacing Congenitally Missing Maxillary Canines and Lateral Incisors

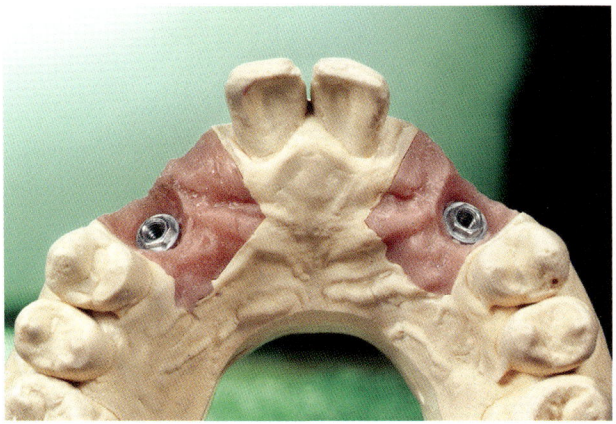

Fig 2-24 Plaster cast with soft tissue simulation: incisal view.

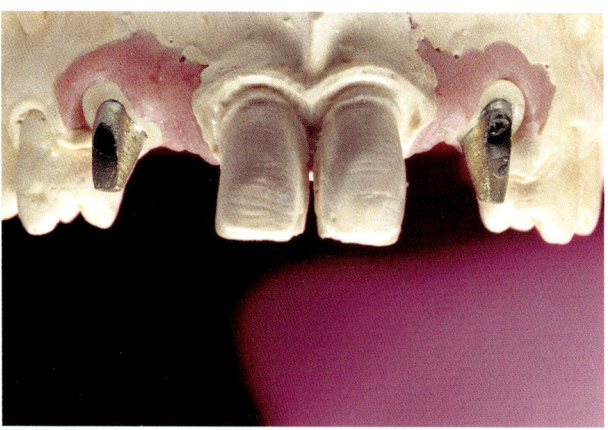

Fig 2-25 Plaster cast with soft tissue simulation and custom fabricated ceramic and gold abutments: anterior view.

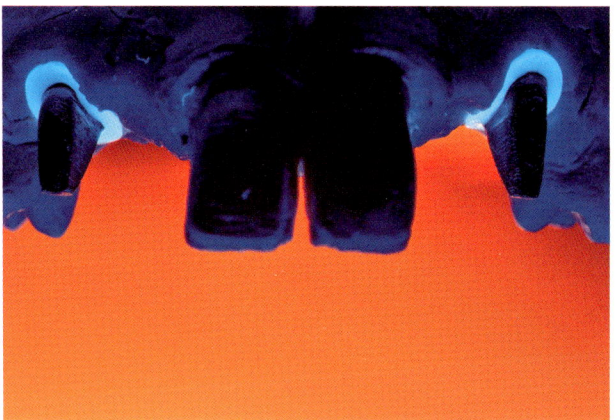

Fig 2-26 Fluorescence of ceramic shoulder porcelain in custom implant abutments.

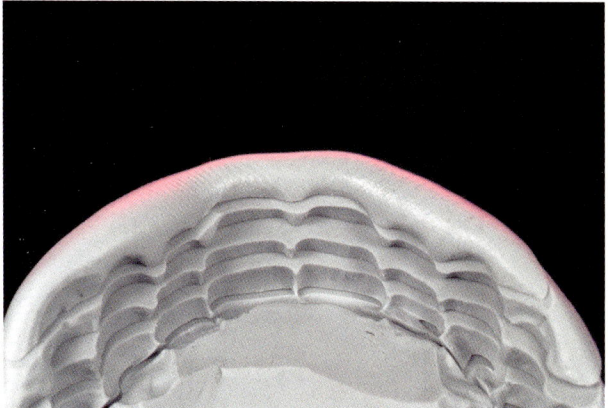

Fig 2-27 Sectioned silicone index, from initial diagnostic waxup, used as a guide for the definitive veneering porcelain buildup.

concave to allow tissue in-growth – an abutment with a convex profile is likely to cause tension of the tissue cuff and possible gingival recession. Another advantage of using an alumina ceramic shoulder is that it gives better light transmission than a titanium abutment, which may appear grayish at the cervical margins because of the thin overlying soft tissues (Fig 2-26).

Using the original diagnostic waxup as a template (Fig 2-11), a silicone index was fabricated and sectioned (Fig 2-27). This served as a guide for the veneering porcelain buildup for creating the anatomical form of the PLVs and cantilever bridges (Figs 2-28 and 2-29).

The completed restorations were as follows (Figs 2-30 and 2-31):
- two custom abutments with screws
- two cement-retained two-unit cantilever bridges
- two PLVs.

2 Replacing Congenitally Missing Maxillary Canines and Lateral Incisors

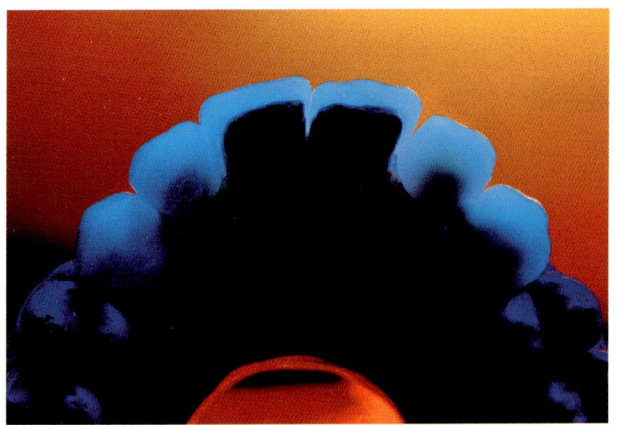

Fig 2-28 Fluorescence of veneering porcelain on definitive restorations.

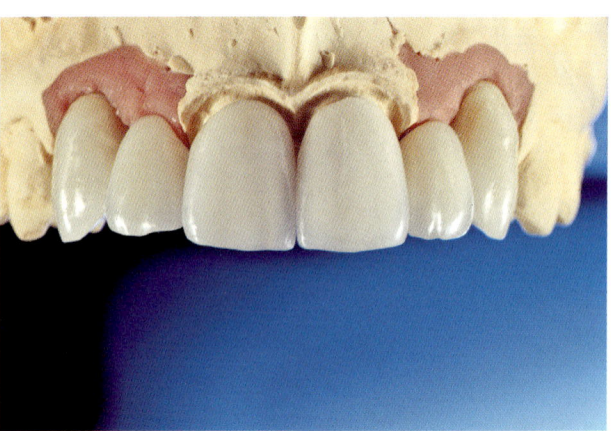

Fig 2-29 Anterior view of completed restorations: two PLVs on centrals and two two-unit cantilever bridges supported by implants at the canine sites.

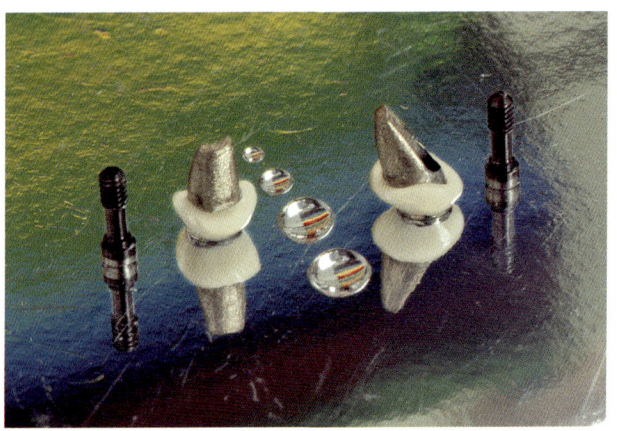

Fig 2-30 Screw-retained custom-fabricated porcelain and gold implant abutments.

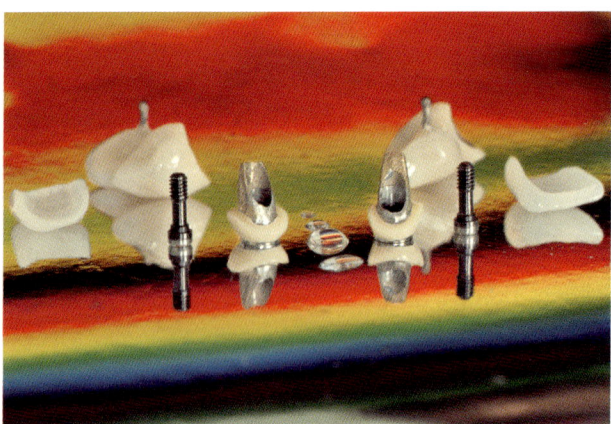

Fig 2-31 Completed restorations consisting of two PLV, two screw-retained abutments, and two cement-retained cantilever bridges.

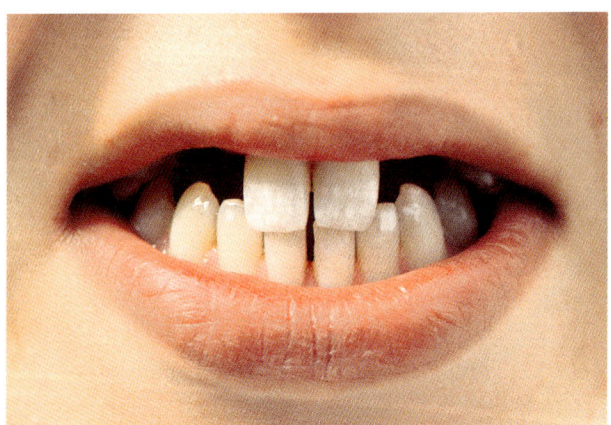

Fig 2-32 Preoperative dento-facial view.

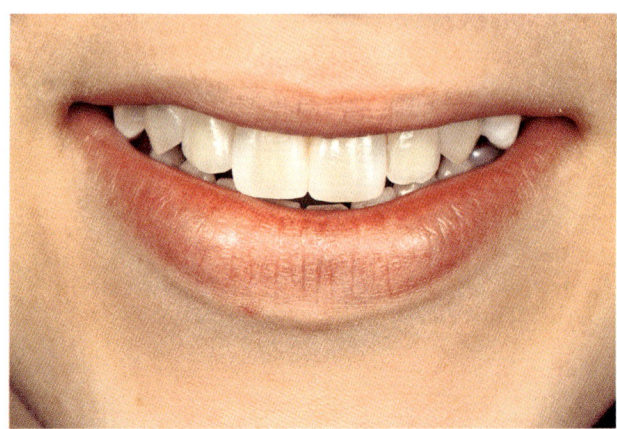

Fig 2-33 Postoperative dento-facial view.

2 Replacing Congenitally Missing Maxillary Canines and Lateral Incisors

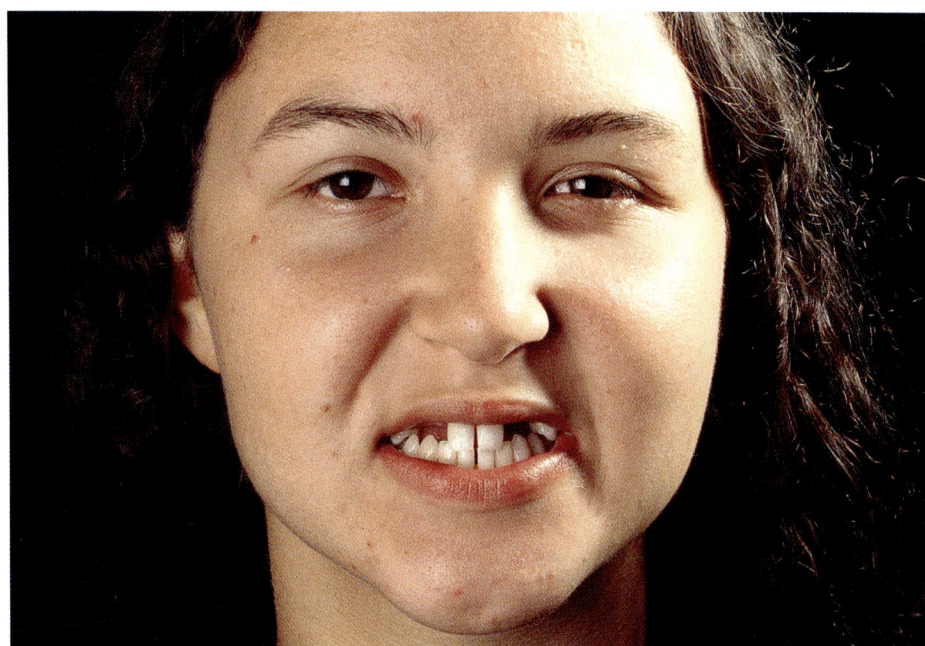

Fig 2-34 Preoperative facial view.

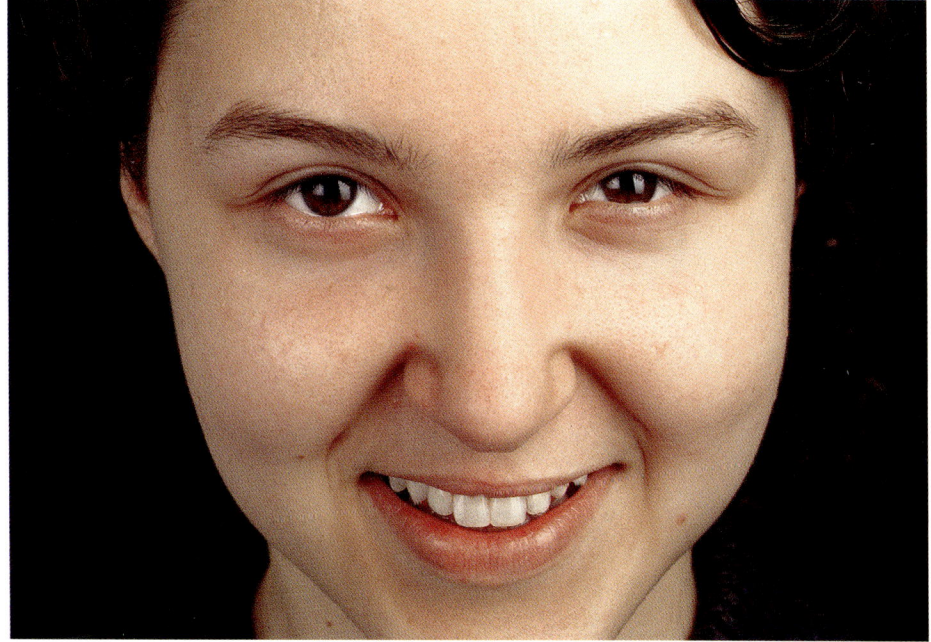

Fig 2-35 Postoperative facial view.

The bridges were cemented with zinc oxide-eugenol cement, and the PLVs with a resin luting agent and a dentin bonding adhesive. Comparison of the preoperative and postoperative views shows restitution of the anterior maxillary sextant (Figs 2-32 to 2-35).

Discussion

There were limitations to the chosen option. First, the thin transmucosal envelope around the canine implant abutments resulted in a poor emergence profile, which was fortunately concealed by the low lip line. Second, during the 5 years following the treatment, both bridges dislodged twice and were subsequently recemented. Although the patient was advised of this possibility, it does prompt the question of whether it would have been prudent to link the implants to the central incisors with FPDs for improved stability.

In hindsight, other options that could have been used to improve the outcome are platelet-rich fibrin to encourage healing, and a locking taper implant design for a hermetic seal or platform switching, which both enhance soft tissue volume around implant abutments. Custom zirconia abutments produced using computer-aided design and computer-assisted manufacture would have negated using cast metal abutments with alumina shoulders. Such an abutment would also have yielded a superior seal with the fixture, especially if the latter were an internal design.

Restoring Structural Integrity and Esthetics Following Tooth Wear

3

Diagnostic waxup and ceramics by Gérald Ubassy, Avignon, France

Pre- and Postoperative Status

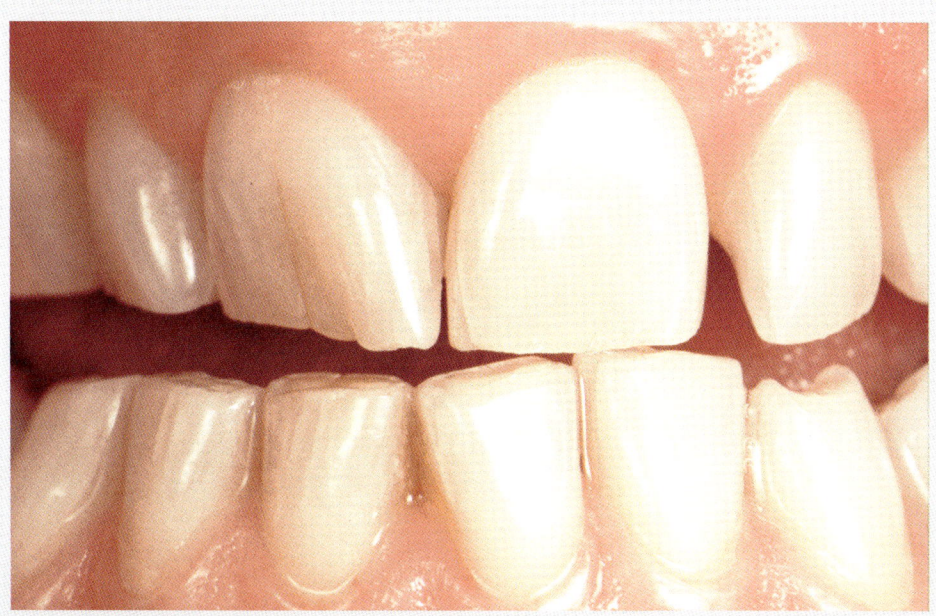

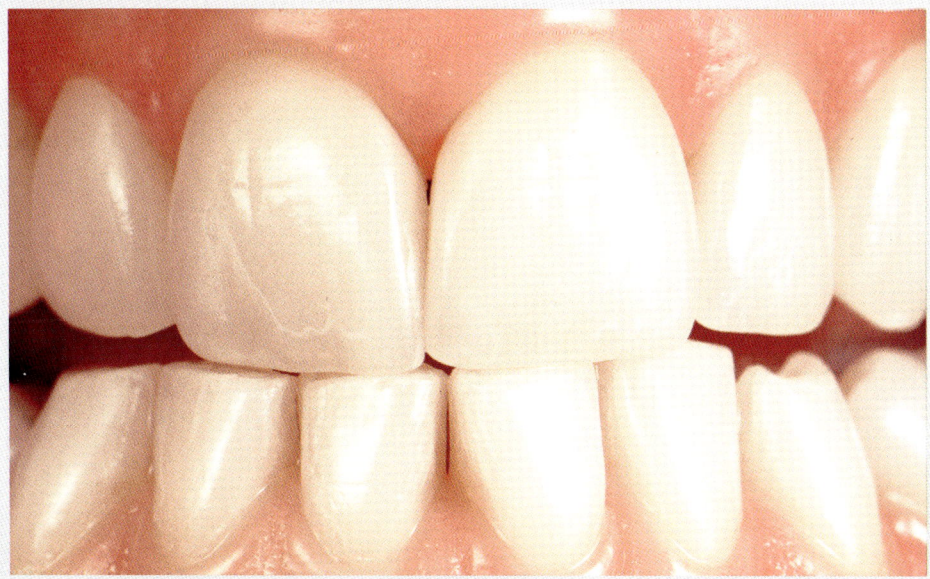

Dental History

A 40-year-old woman, a regular attendee for dental care, requested an improvement of her deteriorating anterior dental esthetics. Ever since her teens, she disliked the diastema between the maxillary left central and lateral incisors and the buccal rotation of the left lateral (Fig 3-1). In addition, tooth wear and discoloration had progressively deteriorated the dentition over the previous 25 years, starting in her twenties (Fig 3-2) and progressing through her thirties (Figs 3-3 and 3-4). Whilst she has endured the wear and staining, she now wished to rectify the problem and halt further destruction to safeguard her dentition (Figs 3-5 and 3-6).

Preoperative Status

Examination revealed tooth wear of mixed etiology: attrition, abrasion, and erosion. Attrition was pronounced on the right maxillary and mandibular canines and incisors (Fig 3-7), resulting in a flattened incisal plane (Figs 3-8 and 3-9). There was also thinning of labial enamel from abrasion, resulting in visibility of the underlying darker dentin strata. The left mandibular canine showed cupping, caused by acidic erosion (Fig 3-10). The diastema and buccal rotation of the left lateral incisor were evident in the left maxillary quadrant (Fig 3-11). The maxillary anterior teeth showed enamel loss at the incisal edges, creating a window of dentin surrounded by intact enamel borders (Fig 3-12).

Treatment Options

1. Ascertain etiology and preventative measures to halt further tooth loss (in preparation for option 2 or option 3).
2. Composite laminate veneers (CLVs) to replace lost enamel and dentin and restore function and esthetics.
3. Porcelain laminate veneers (PLVs) to replace lost enamel and dentin and restore function and esthetics.

Scientific Credence for Treatment Options

Tooth wear is non-carious destruction and loss of tooth substrate, primarily a result of lifestyle choices. Examples include stress-induced grinding habits (attrition), eating and drinking acidic foods and effervescent drinks (erosion), and toothpaste abuse (abrasion). Initial management of tooth loss, therefore, involves counseling and oral hygiene instruction, followed by repair or replacement of the lost tooth substrate.

Methods for treating lost enamel and dentin include bleaching, occlusal splints, composite fillings, PLVs, and full-coverage crowns. The method used will depend on the degree of loss. The choice for this case study was between composite and porcelain veneers (options 2 and 3). A comparison of these two modalities is shown in Table 3-1.

3 Restoring Structural Integrity and Esthetics Following Tooth Wear

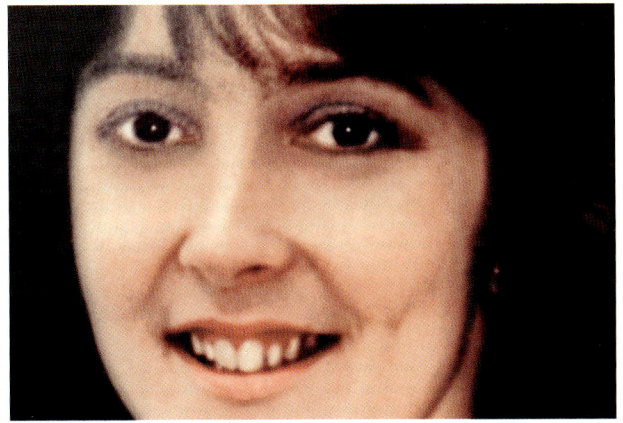
Fig 3-1 Patient in her teens.

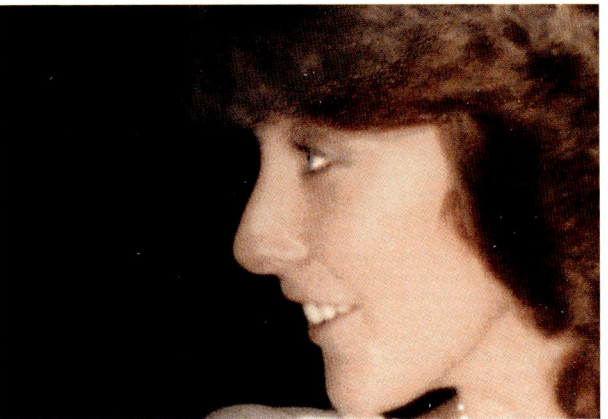
Fig 3-2 Patient in her twenties.

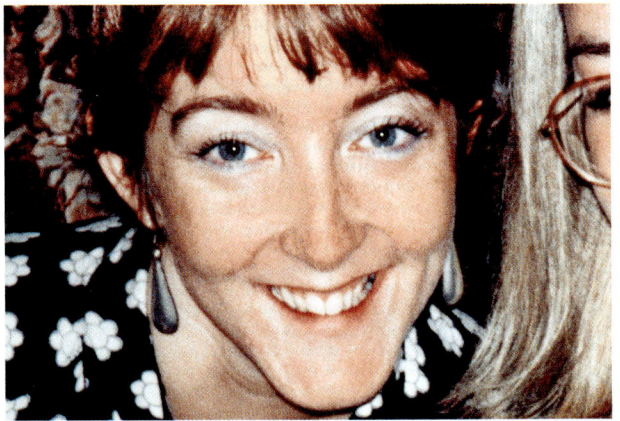
Fig 3-3 Patient in her thirties.

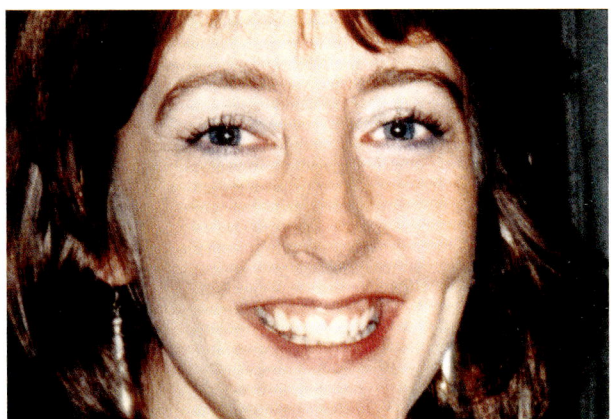
Fig 3-4 Patient in her thirties.

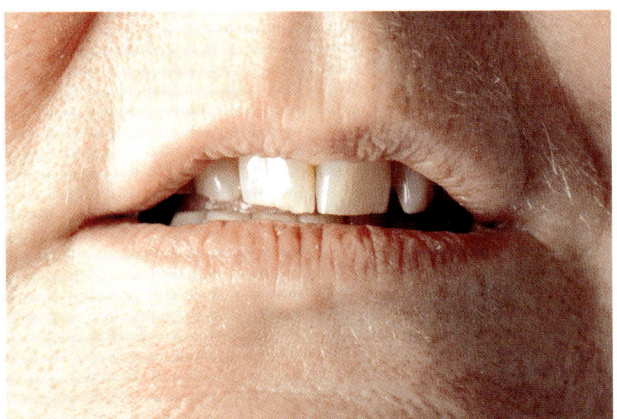
Fig 3-5 Preoperative dento-facial view, showing degree of tooth exposure at rest.

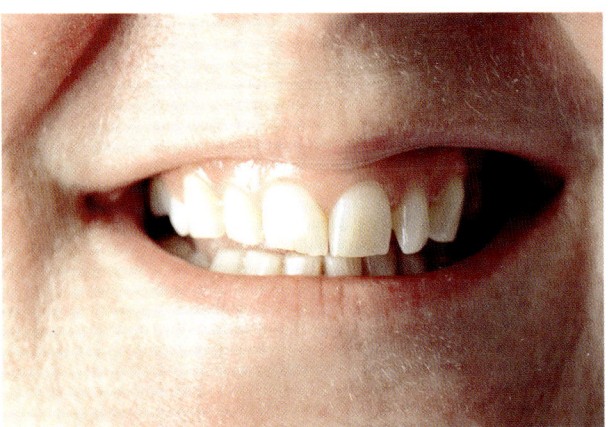
Fig 3-6 Preoperative dento-facial view, showing degree of tooth exposure during a relaxed smile.

3 Restoring Structural Integrity and Esthetics Following Tooth Wear

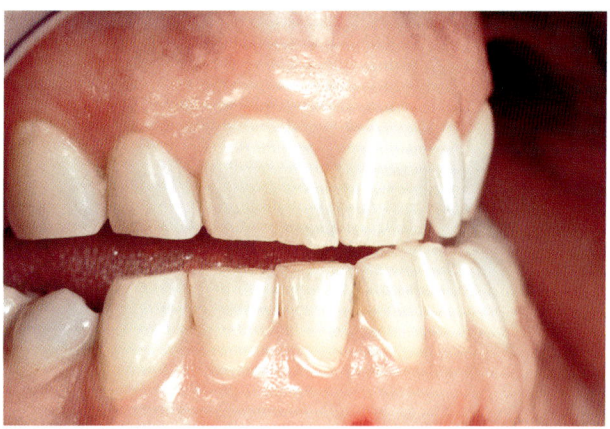

Fig 3-7 Preoperative right lateral view showing worn, flattened incisal plane.

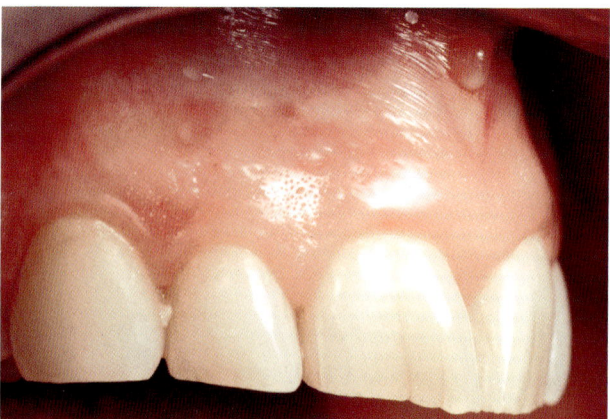

Fig 3-8 Preoperative right lateral view showing flattened incisal plane.

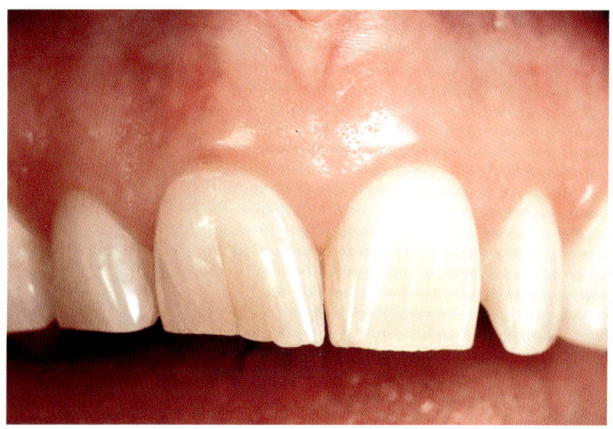

Fig 3-9 Preoperative anterior view showing incisal edge wear.

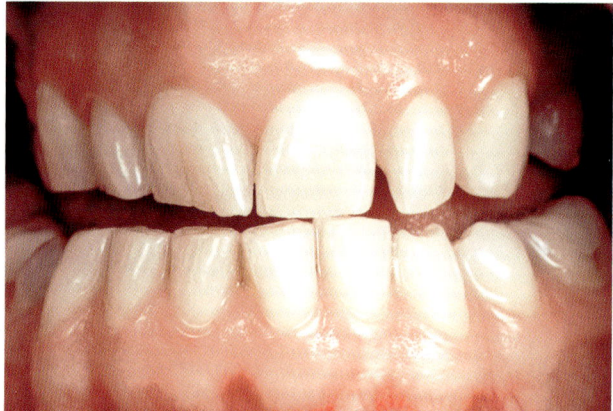

Fig 3-10 Preoperative left lateral view showing rotation of the left lateral and incisal cupping of the left mandibular canine caused by acidic erosion.

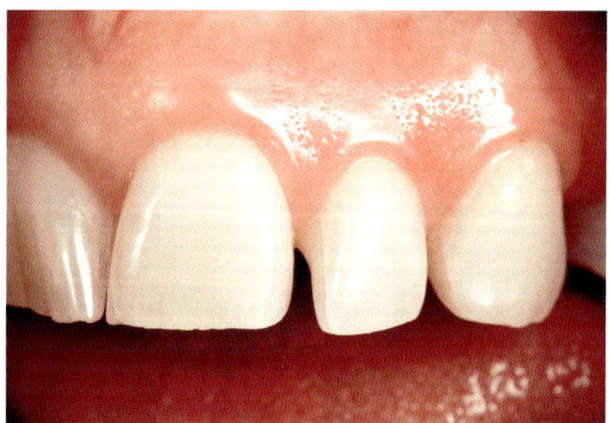

Fig 3-11 Detailed view of diastema and buccal rotation of left lateral incisor.

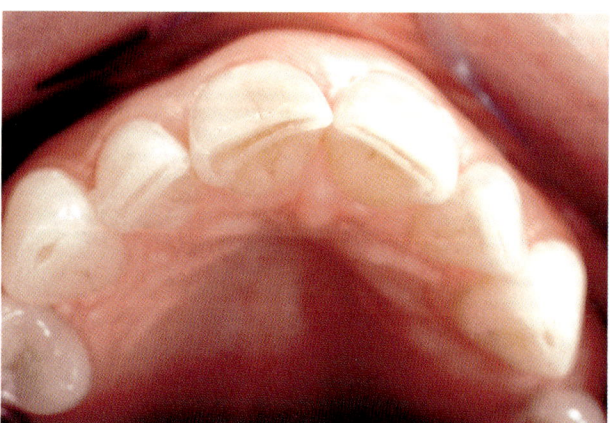

Fig 3-12 Incisal edge wear of maxillary incisors and canines.

Composite laminate veneers	Porcelain laminate veneers
Susceptible to wear and deformation	Resistant to wear, retains form
Chromatically unstable	Chromatically stable
Marginal fractures	Fractures of ceramics likely with poor laboratory and clinical protocols
Do not restore tooth rigidity (elastic modulus of microfilled hybrid composite is 10–20 GPa)	Restore tooth rigidity (elastic modulus of 80 GPa is similar to enamel overlay)
Increase plaque accumulation	Reduce plaque accumulation
	Superior optical properties, ability to incorporate characteristics such as translucencies, mamelons, etc.
	Precipitate antagonist natural tooth wear in bruxists

Table 3-1 Comparison of composite and porcelain laminate veneers.

Clinical Erudition and Feasibility

Patient counseling and monitoring of tooth wear are essential for prevention of enamel or dentin loss. The points to consider before selecting CLVs or PLVs are as follows. Both options are technique sensitive, requiring knowledge about adhesive protocols and dentin-bonding agents. CLVs are time consuming and require a degree of dexterity and patience, but they do not require the use of a ceramist or a second visit for luting. PLVs can produce superlative esthetics, but to achieve this the ceramist should not only have technical competence but also possess artistic flair. Of course, the use of a dental laboratory and the second visit for luting means PLVs are more expensive for the patient.

Patient Needs and Wants

Adherence to an oral hygiene regimen and dietary advice is prerequisite before commencing reparative treatment. Also, compliance with a nightguard or mouth guard is essential to mitigate grinding habits and protect replacement restorations.

If the patient wants a quick fix, with acceptable esthetics, lower cost, and faster treatment, CLVs are the treatment of choice. However, the patient must understand that regular maintenance is required and replacement may be necessary owing to staining and wear of the resin composite. If cost is not a constraint and superlative esthetics are a priority, PLVs are the ideal choice, but the treatment time will be lengthy. In this case, the patient opted for PLVs.

Treatment Sequence

The chosen treatment option was six PLVs for the maxillary canines and incisors. PLVs are extensively used, and abused, for esthetic and cosmetic dentistry. The dictum to remember before prescribing these restorations is:
- PLVs are for replacing lost enamel and dentin
- PLVs are NOT a substitute for enamel and dentin.

If the above is followed, PLVs can be, and indeed are, a very predictable and successful treatment modality.

The first stage is to carry out a shade analysis to determine the prevailing tooth discoloration and the feasibility of the desired shade (Fig 3-13). This is followed by a diagnostic waxup to ascertain the amount of lost tooth substrate requiring replacement (Figs 3-14 to 3-17). The waxup has many uses, including composite resin mock-up veneers (Fig 3-18), silicone indices in various planes (eg, bucco-lingual, sagittal), and transparent vacuum stents for fabricating provisional restorations (Fig 3-19). All, or some of these items are invaluable for diagnosis, assessment, and patient satisfaction before proceeding to tooth preparation.

Unlike full-coverage crowns, for PLVs there is no ideal tooth preparation. Tooth reduction, if necessary, is dictated by the extent of tooth loss, treatment aims and objectives (eg, masking underlying tooth discoloration), and the type of ceramic to be used. Tooth reduction for PLVs involves four aspects: buccal reduction, incisal edge reduction, cervical margins, and interproximal contacts (Figs 3-20 and 3-21).

Buccal Reduction

Buccal reduction is almost exclusively determined by silicone indices of the diagnostic waxup, but the following guidelines should be observed (Fig 3-22).
- Assess the amount of remaining tooth substrate (larger pulps and thick enamel in youth, and smaller pulps, secondary dentin, and reduced enamel overlay in people over 50 years of age).
- There must be sufficient thickness for the chosen ceramic system (especially for bite collapse as a consequence of tooth wear and alveolar compensation), eg, unilayer ceramic systems, 0.3 mm for the cervical one-third and 0.5 mm for the incisal two-thirds; and bilayer ceramic systems, 0.5 mm for the cervical one-third and 0.7 mm for the incisal two-thirds.
- Preparation should be smooth, devoid of undercuts.
- Preparation should be non-uniform, ie, less reduction in cervical areas where enamel overlay is thin or absent.
- Ensure two-thirds to three-quarters of the enamel thickness should remain to preserve tooth rigidity and achieve superior enamel bonding.
- Debonding is more likely when the exposed dentin surface area is greater than 80%.

3 Restoring Structural Integrity and Esthetics Following Tooth Wear

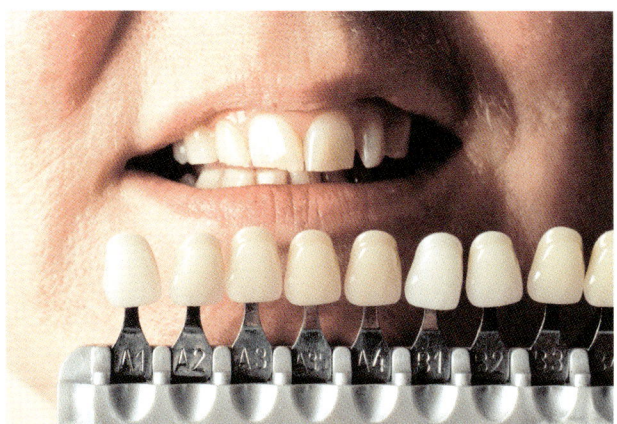

Fig 3-13 Shade analysis with Vita Classical shade guide.

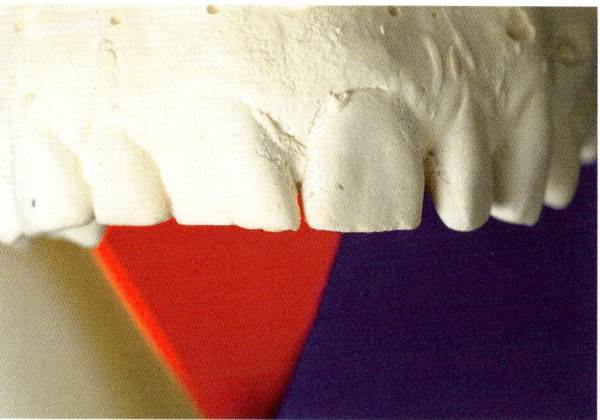

Fig 3-14 Preoperative plaster cast: anterior view.

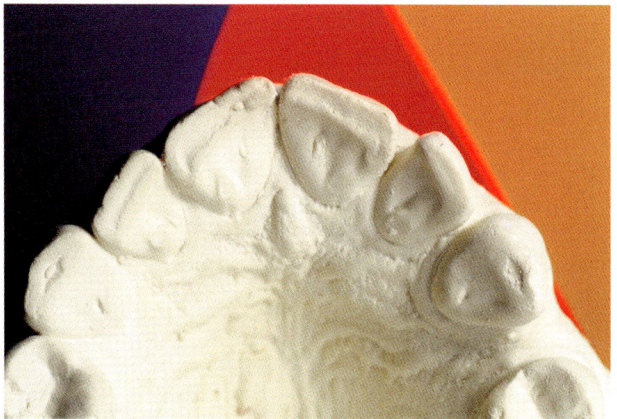

Fig 3-15 Preoperative plaster cast: incisal view.

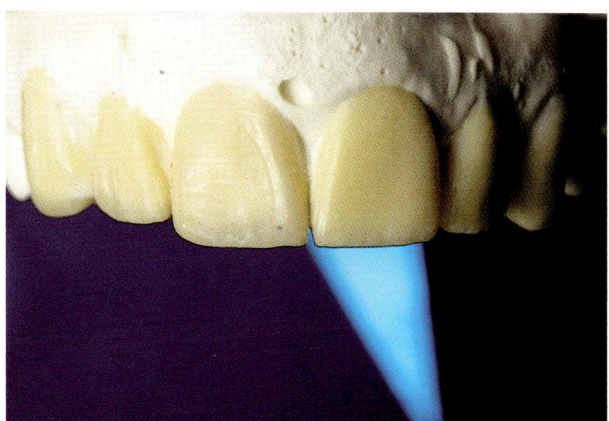

Fig 3-16 Diagnostic waxup: anterior view.

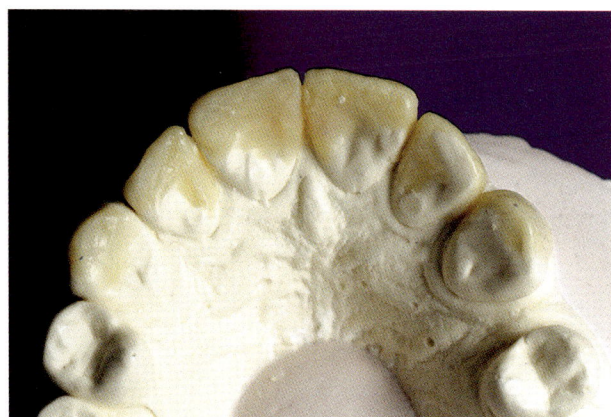

Fig 3-17 Diagnostic wax-up: incisal view.

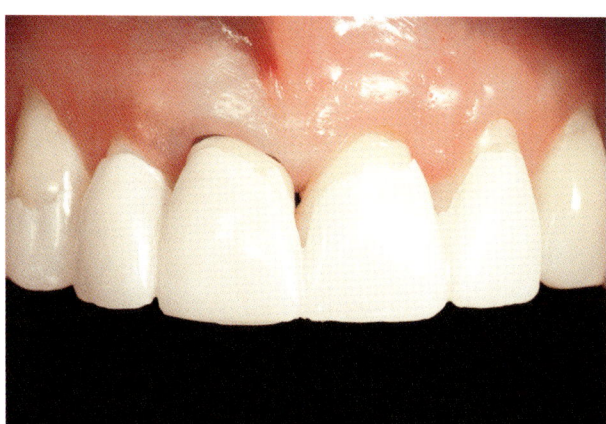

Fig 3-18 Resin composite mock-up of proposed restorations.

27

3 Restoring Structural Integrity and Esthetics Following Tooth Wear

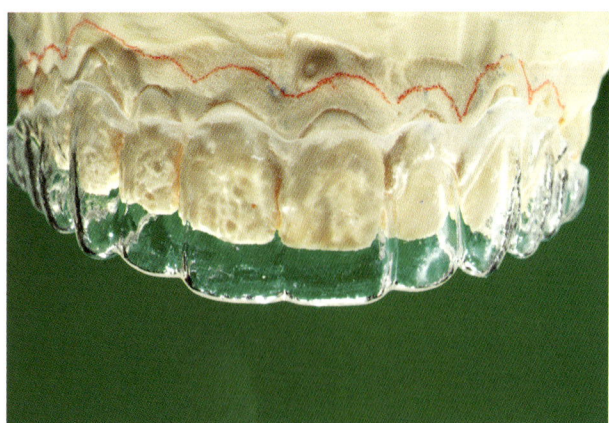
Fig 3-19 Transparent vacuum stent from diagnostic waxup for fabrication of chairside provisional restorations.

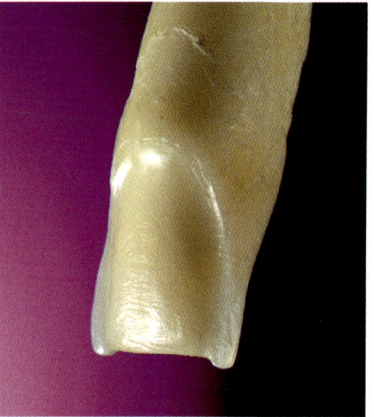
Fig 3-20 Anterior lateral view of PLV preparation on a maxillary incisor.

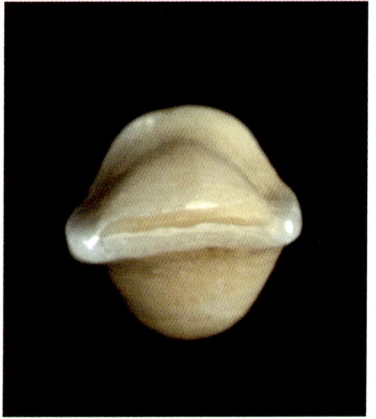
Fig 3-21 Incisal view of PLV preparation on a maxillary incisor.

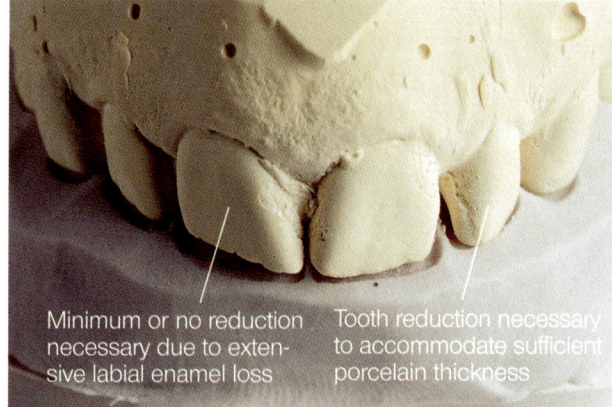
Fig 3-22 Silicone index from diagnostic waxup dictating the amount of tooth reduction necessary for PLVs.

Bearing the above in mind, tooth preparation can be accomplished using a variety of rotary instruments. Uniform depth gauges are contraindicated since tooth reduction is identical at the cervical and incisal aspects (Fig 3-23). This results in excessive enamel removal at the cervical aspects, which have very thin or no enamel and, therefore, the exposure of dentin is inevitable. The ideal burs are either individual depth gauges of varying diameters (Fig 3-24), or round burs (Fig 3-25), again of different diameters, for selective reduction at the cervical and incisal aspects. The buccal reduction is completed by joining the depth cuts using a tapered chamfer bur (Fig 3-26), which also creates the cervical margin (discussed below).

Incisal Edge Reduction

There are four types of incisal edge reduction: window, feather-edge, palatal bevel, and palatal chamfer. The window (Fig 3-27) and feather-edge (Fig 3-28)

3 Restoring Structural Integrity and Esthetics Following Tooth Wear

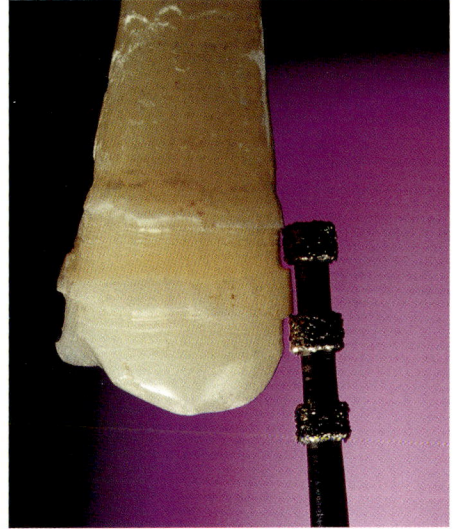

Fig 3-23 Buccal reduction for PLVs: using a uniform depth gauge.

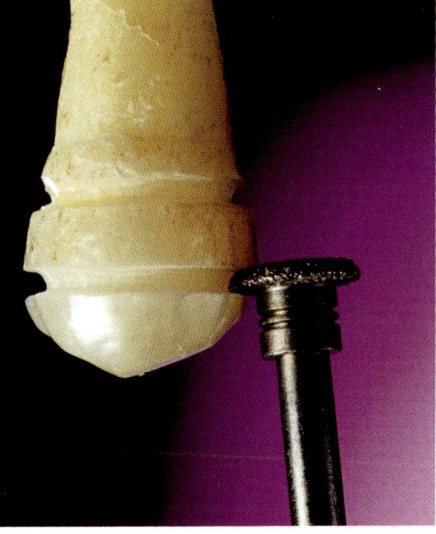

Fig 3-24 Buccal reduction for PLVs: using disc.

Fig 3-25 Buccal reduction for PLVs: using round burs of different diameters.

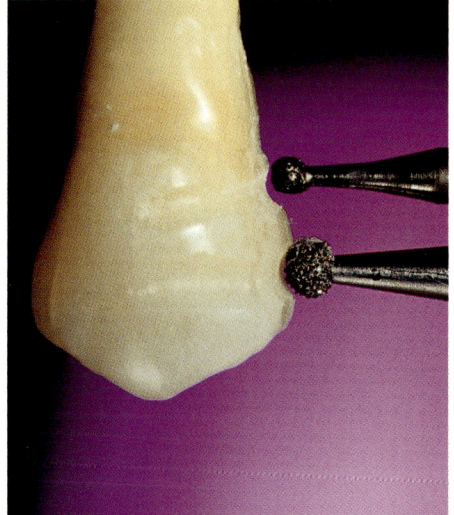

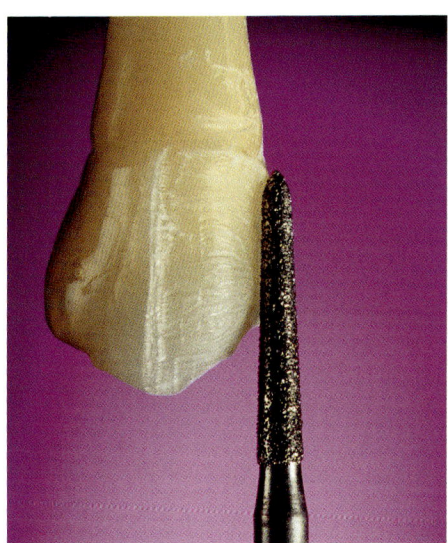

Fig 3-26 Buccal reduction for PLVs: using a tapered chamfer bur.

reductions are minimally invasive, retaining the original length and incisal edge of the tooth. However, their drawbacks are possible chipping at the incisal edges and visibility of the cement line (especially if the cement line becomes discolored), and they are inappropriate for tooth lengthening. The palatal bevel (Fig 3-29) and palatal chamfer (Fig 3-30) both permit tooth lengthening, better incisal esthetics, alteration of the incisal edge shape, and positive seating at the try-in and luting stages. Their drawback is the invasive preparation, requiring 1.5–2 mm occlusal clearance. The literature states that the survival rate of PLVs using any of these incisal edge preparations is identical. Therefore, the ultimate choice depends on the clinical situation and the aims and objectives of treatment. The last point to consider is the location of the palatal finish line. The finish line should avoid centric contacts and the palatal concavity, which is the area of maximum stress concentration (Fig 3-31).

3 Restoring Structural Integrity and Esthetics Following Tooth Wear

Fig 3-27 Incisal edge reduction for PLVs: window.

Fig 3-28 Incisal edge reduction for PLVs: feather edge.

Fig 3-29 Incisal edge reduction for PLVs: palatal bevel.

Fig 3-30 Incisal edge reduction for PLVs: palatal chamfer.

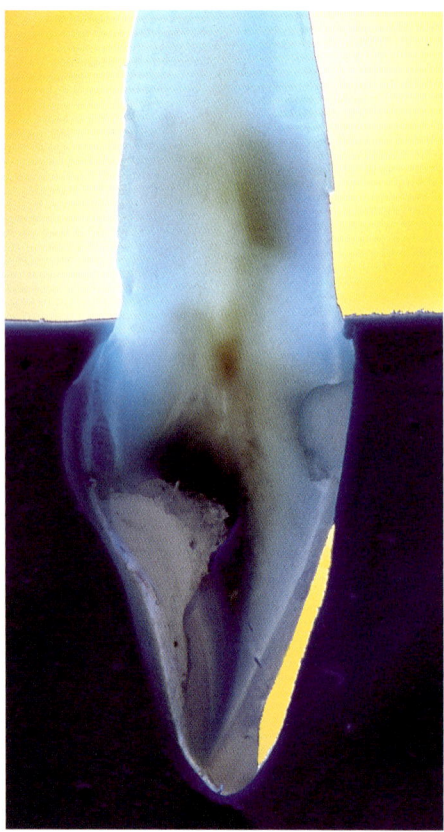
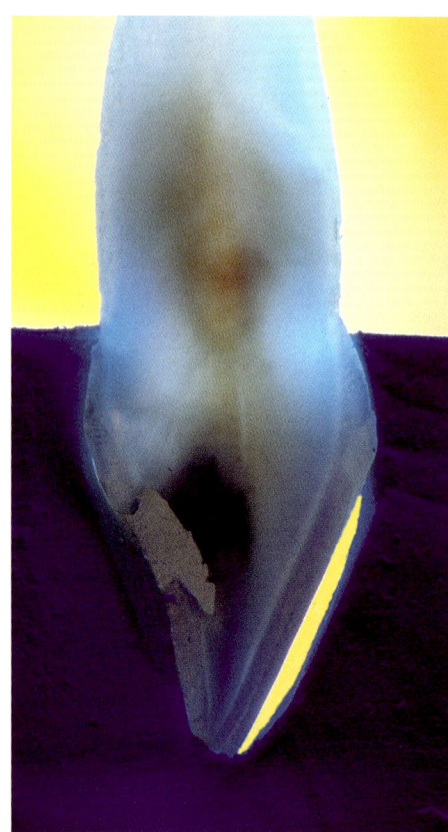
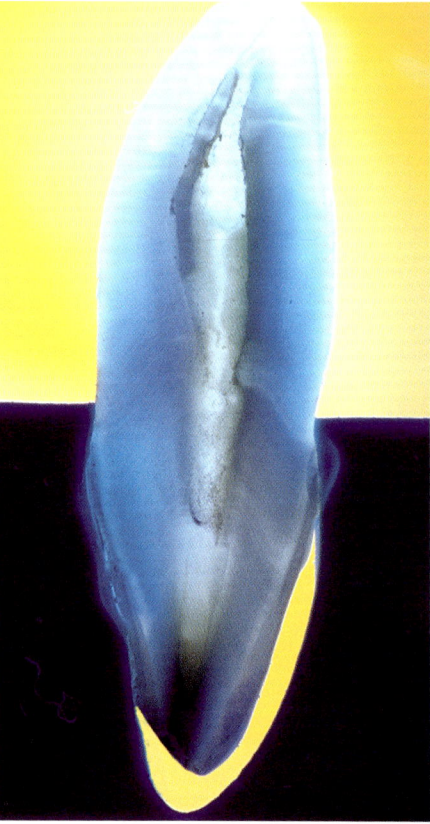
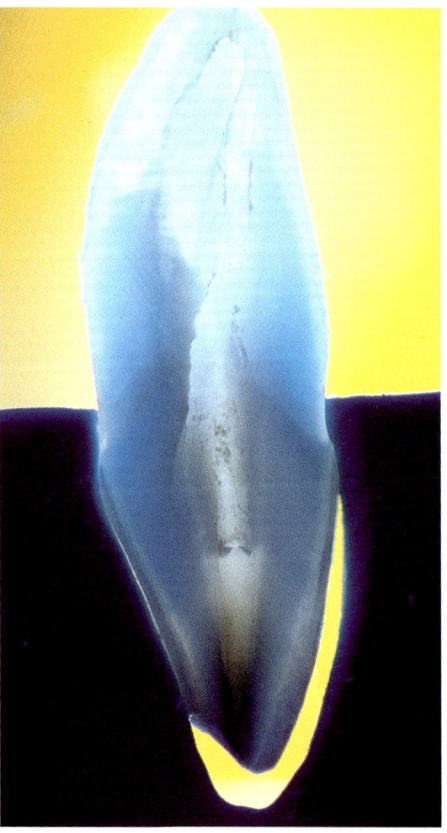

3 Restoring Structural Integrity and Esthetics Following Tooth Wear

Cervical Margins

The cervical margins can be placed supra-, equi-, or subgingivally. Supra- or equigingival margins are indicated for a low lip line or a thin dental biotype (Fig 3-32). Subgingival margins are reserved for a high lip line, to mask profound discoloration, or when using dense ceramic cores, but only with a thick dental biotype (Fig 3-33).

Interproximal Contacts

There are two opinions regarding breaking or retaining interproximal contact points. The arguments for retaining contacts are to prevent unwanted tooth movement during the temporization period and to retain maximum tooth structure. The opposing view is to break contacts 1 mm palatally, which facilitates impression making, fabrication and cementation procedures as well as concealing the cement line. The principles for either are debatable, and the choice will depend on the clinician's experience and clinical judgment.

The completed preparations possess the following features:
- healthy, free gingival margins
- subgingival margin location (for thick biotype)
- where possible, tooth reduction confined to enamel; notice bur marks that are located within the enamel (Figs 3-34 and 3-35)
- broken contact points
- immediate sealing of exposed dentin: necessary with the bucally rotated left lateral incisor (Fig 3-36)
- minimal incisal reduction owing to existing enamel loss at the incisal edges (Fig 3-37)
- smooth line angles, devoid of undercuts
- palatal chamfer, avoiding centric contact and palatal concavity.

Impressions were made using silicone impression material with a low contact angle, addition (Panasil, Kettenbach, Germany) (Fig 3-38). Any loose retraction cord was trimmed, but tenaciously embedded cord was left in situ until the plaster model was cast (Fig 3-39). This prevented tearing the finish lines of the

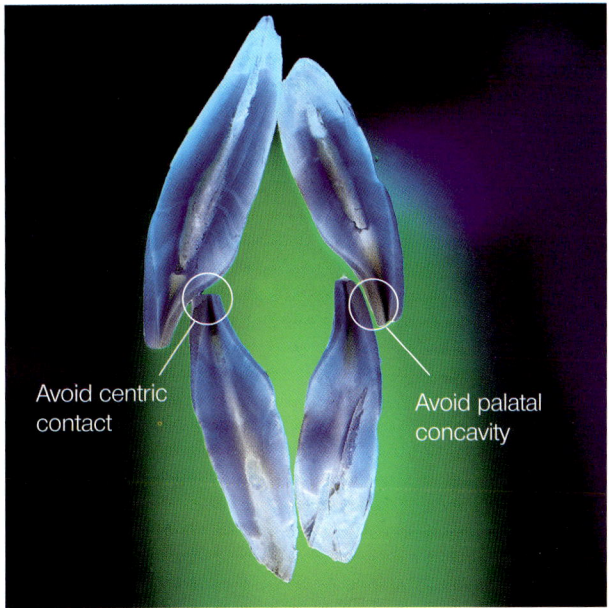

Fig 3-31 Incisal edge reduction for PLVs: avoid incisal contact and palatal concavity.

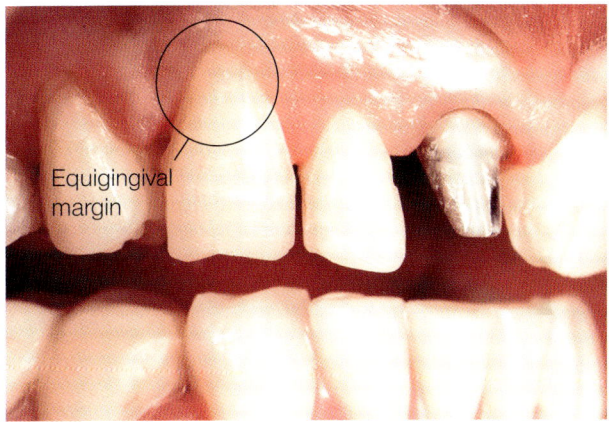

Fig 3-32 Cervical margin for PLVs: equigingival location.

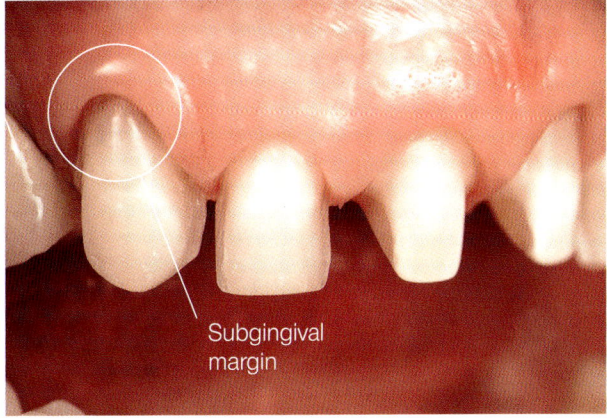

Fig 3-33 Cervical margin for PLVs: subgingival location.

3 Restoring Structural Integrity and Esthetics Following Tooth Wear

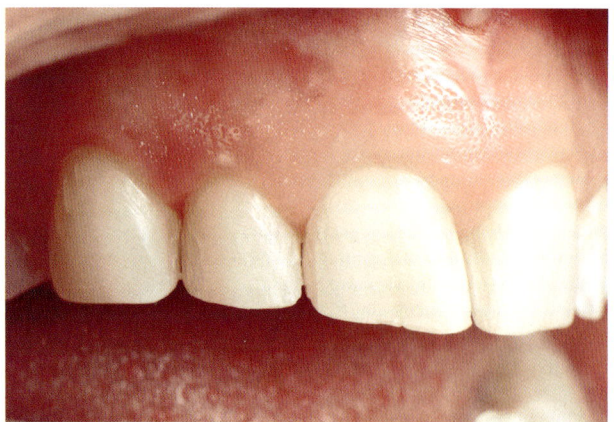

Fig 3-34 Completed PLV preparations: right lateral view.

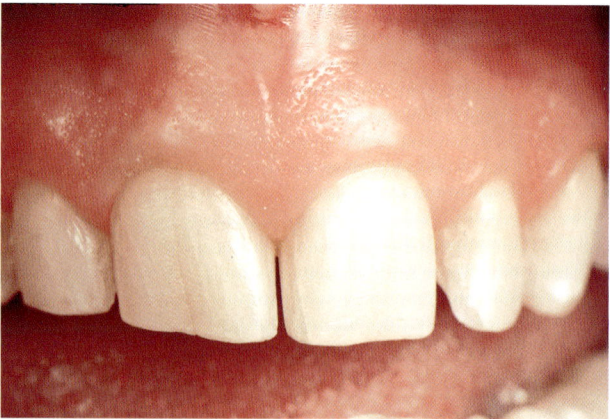

Fig 3-35 Completed PLV preparations: anterior view.

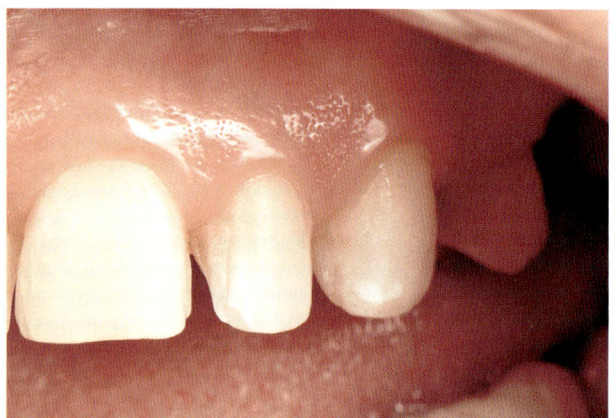

Fig 3-36 Completed PLV preparations: left lateral view.

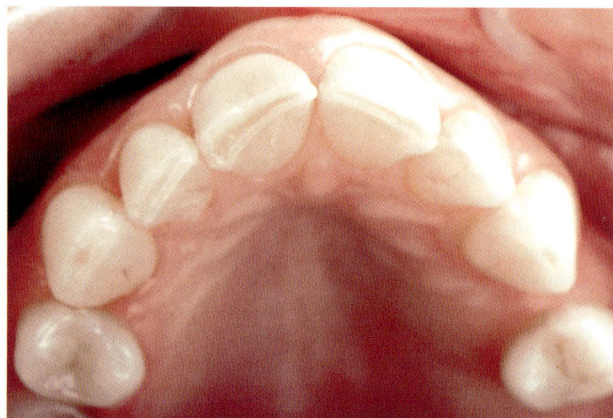

Fig 3-37 Completed PLV preparations: incisal view.

tooth preparation. The plaster casts show a faithful reproduction of the preparations, including the bur marks (which were confined to the enamel layer) (Figs 3-40 and 3-41). Areas apical to the finish line were captured and subsequently trimmed, allowing the ceramist to create correct emergence profiles, and the palatal finish lines were delineated with red pencil marks (Fig 3-42).

The final factor to consider for PLV is the luting agent. The ideal luting agents for cementing PLVs are resin-based cements, which can either be light cured or dual cured (in conjunction with silane pretreatment of the intaglio surface), or the latest self-adhesive varieties, which do not require silane pretreatment. Compared with zinc phosphate and glass–ionomer cements, resin-based cements offer a number of advantages. These include improved rigidity of the tooth/cement/veneer complex and suitability for all types of ceramic material. With silica-based ceramics, resin-based cements offer either micromechanical retention on the intaglio surface or chemical coupling in conjunction with saline. With

3 Restoring Structural Integrity and Esthetics Following Tooth Wear

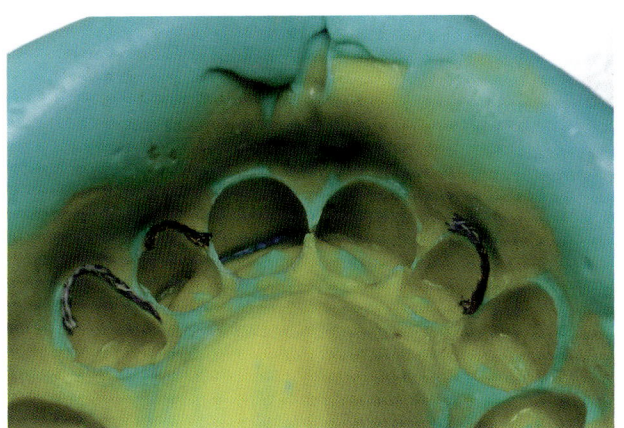

Fig 3-38 Impression of PLV preparations: incisal view.

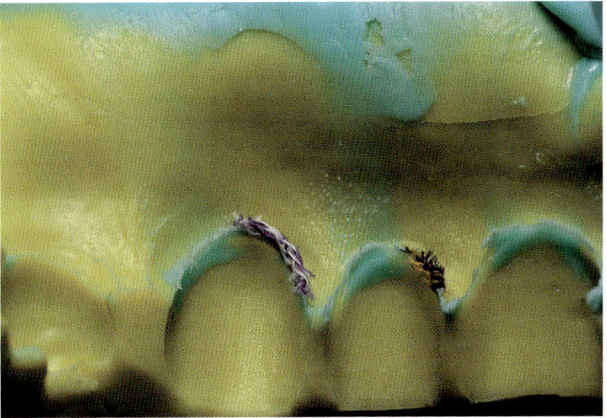

Fig 3-39 Impression of PLV preparations: buccal view.

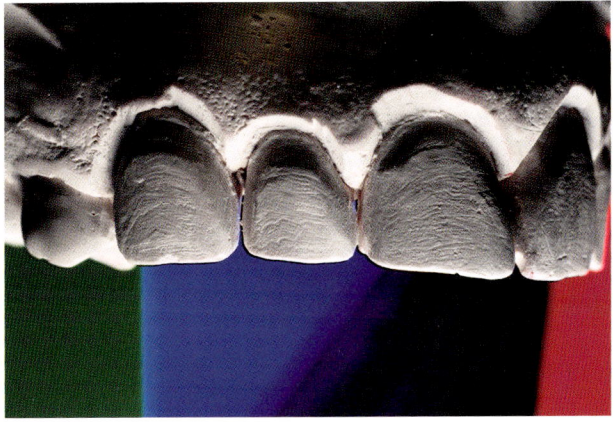

Fig 3-40 Plaster cast of PLV preparations: right lateral view.

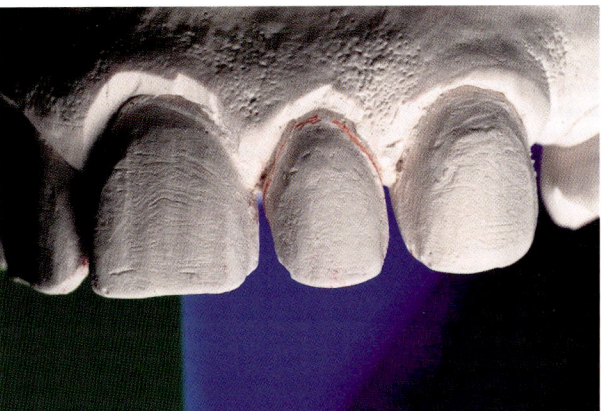

Fig 3-41 Plaster cast of PLV preparations: left lateral view.

alumina- or zirconia-based ceramics, self-adhesive varieties containing an adhesive phosphate monomer (methacryloyloxydecyl dihydrogen phosphate; MDP) offer chemical adhesion on the intaglio surface. Other advantages are polymerization shrinkage. While this is detrimental for direct composite fillings, it is advantageous for luting because the shrinkage "heals" or seals flaws on the intaglio surface.

Pretreatment of the intaglio surface is determined by the type of ceramic. For dense ceramics (alumina and zirconia based), air particle abrasion is the ideal choice. However, for the weaker silica-based ceramics, air abrasion may fracture and chip the delicate porcelain, especially at the

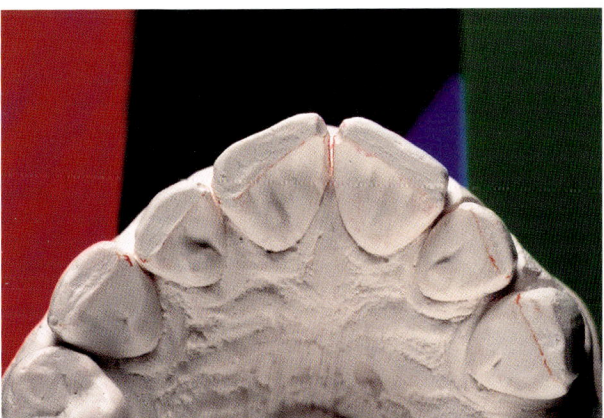

Fig 3-42 Plaster cast of PLV preparations: incisal view.

3 Restoring Structural Integrity and Esthetics Following Tooth Wear

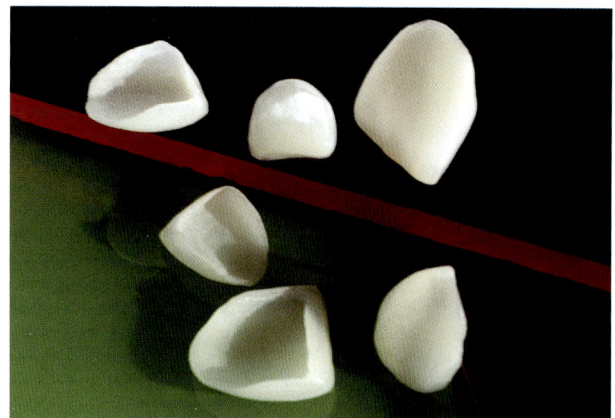

Fig 3-43 Completed PLV restaurations.

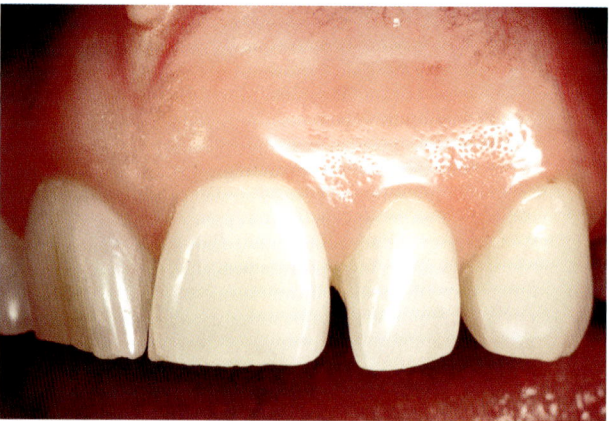

Fig 3-44 Left lateral preoperative view.

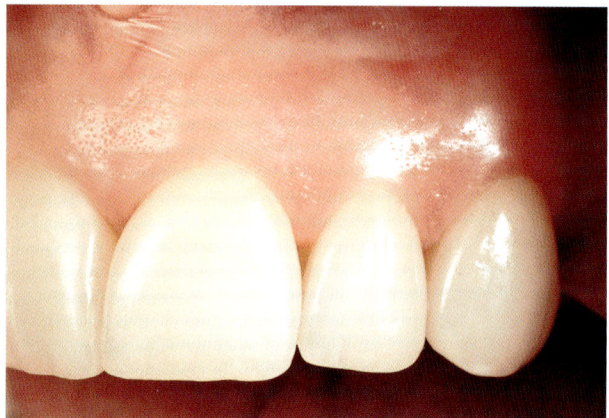

Fig 3-45 Left lateral postoperative view.

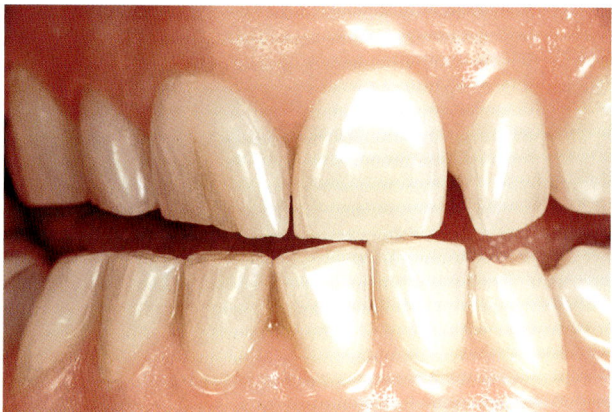

Fig 3-46 Anterior preoperative view.

margins, and hydrofluoric acid is therefore a better option (Fig 3-43). Caution is necessary when using hydrofluoric acid, as prolonged exposure may weaken or dissolve the intaglio surface, thus defeating the object of roughening the surface to increase mechanical retention.

The silica-based PLVs were luted with resin-based cement using hydrofluoric acid and a silane coupling agent. The left lateral pre- and postoperative views show impeccable integration of the PLVs with the surrounding periodontium and elimination of the diastema and buccal rotation of the left lateral incisor (Figs 3-44 and 3-45). The anterior (Figs 3-46 and 3-47) and incisal

3 Restoring Structural Integrity and Esthetics Following Tooth Wear

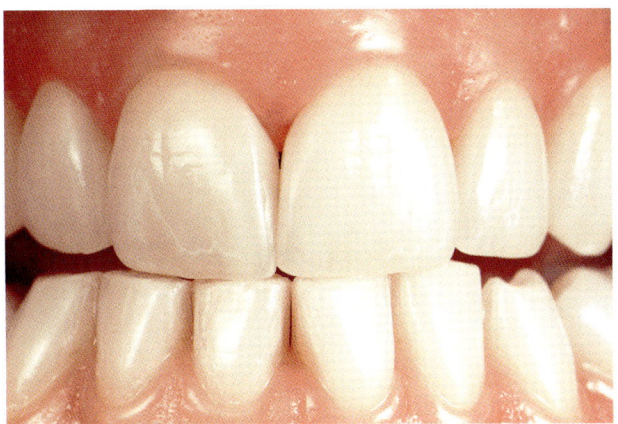

Fig 3-47 Anterior postoperative view.

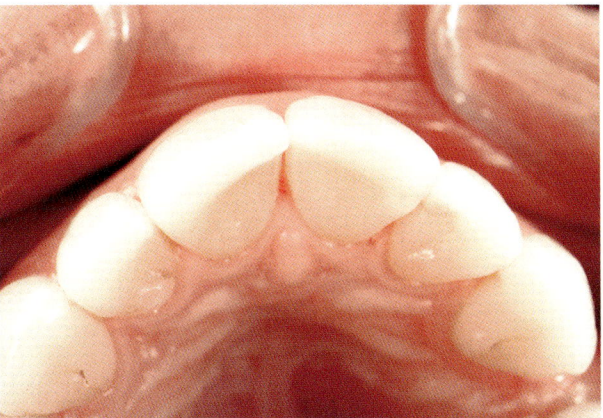

Fig 3-48 Incisal postoperative view.

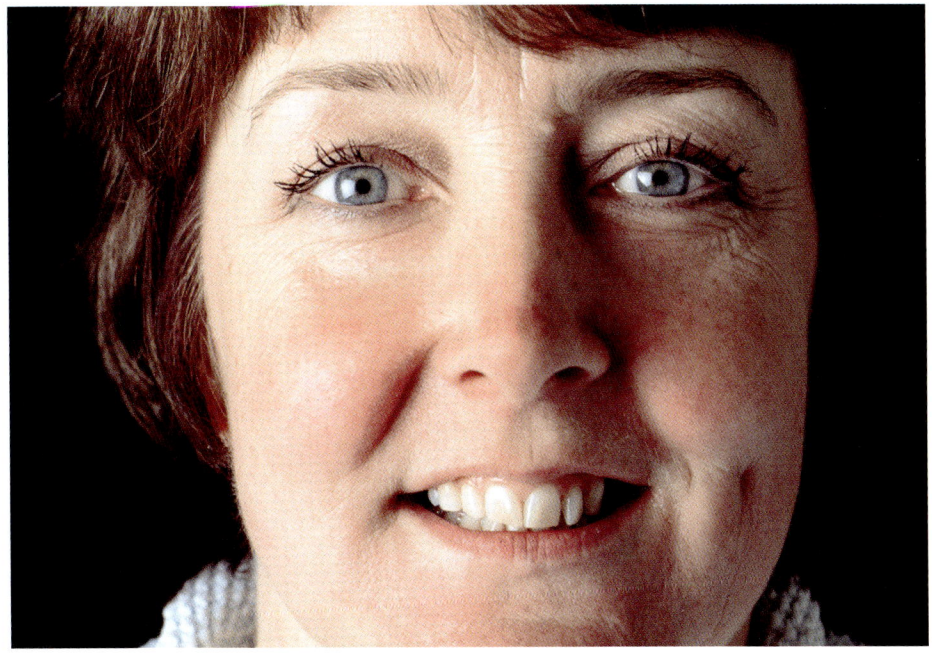

Fig 3-49 Preoperative frontal facial view.

(Fig 3-48) views show replacement of the lost enamel by the PLVs and restitution of anterior esthetics. The preoperative (Fig 3-49) and postoperative facial views (Fig 3-50 and 3-51) reinforce the esthetic improvement and the achievement of the initial objectives of the treatment: to restore health, function, and esthetics, and to safeguard against further tooth wear.

3 Restoring Structural Integrity and Esthetics Following Tooth Wear

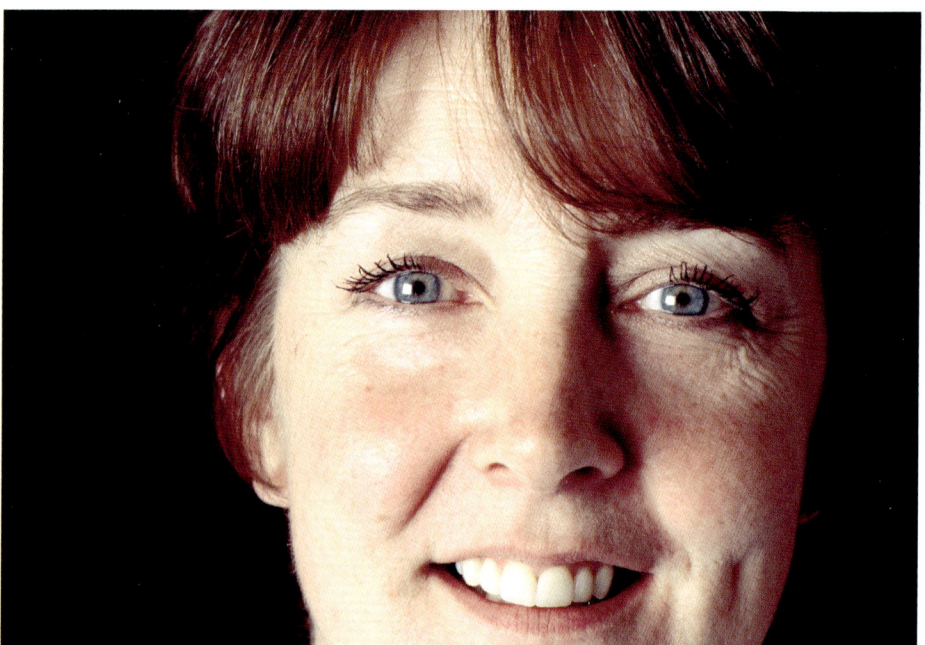

Fig 3-50 Postoperative frontal facial view.

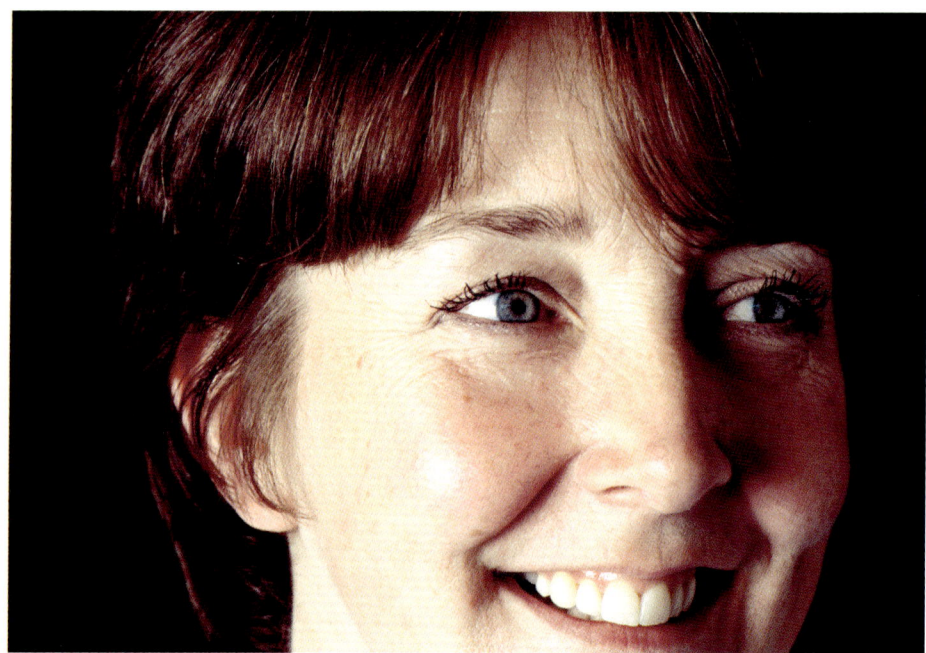

Fig 3-51 Postoperative right frontal facial view.

Discussion

Regular assessment is essential to monitor tooth wear, and oral hygiene and dietary advice should be periodically reinforced. In addition, a nightguard is helpful for mitigating grinding habits and retarding attrition.

Restoring the mandibular arch is more complex. The incisal cupping from acidic erosion can be easily sealed with direct composite fillings. However, because of alveolar compensation, there is insufficient space to accommodate restorative materials to restore the incisors. Two methods are available to create interocclusal clearance. The first is to reposition the mandible in centric relation using an anterior deprogrammer. The principle of this is that, during wear, the mandible moves in an anterior and superior direction. The anterior deprogrammer (eg, Lucia jig) helps to locate the mandible in centric relation, thereby repositioning it in a posterior and inferior direction, creating the necessary space for the restorative materials. The second method is to use an anterior Dahl appliance to allow periodontal eruption of the posterior teeth. Once the posterior occlusion is stable, and sufficient space created anteriorly, the mandibular incisors can be restored using PLVs in a similar manner to the anterior maxillary teeth.

Another possible scenario is where simultaneous wear of both anterior and posterior teeth has occurred. In these circumstances, a less-destructive option compared with full-coverage crowns is to place onlays on to the posterior teeth (to increase the vertical dimension of occlusion) and PLVs on the incisors. The more invasive approach of full-coverage restorations on the posterior teeth to "open the bite" should be resisted, because removing further enamel and dentin from a tooth already compromised by wear will only weaken it further.

Finally, if discoloration is profound and cannot be masked by unilayer ceramics, bilayer PLVs can be considered. The bilayer systems have dense cores that are veneered with a second, superficial porcelain layer. For example, a Procera laminate (Nobel Biocare, Sweden) consists of a 0.25 mm alumina substructure that is veneered with a 0.45 mm layer of porcelain. The benefit is that the dense core has greater masking capabilities, but the system requires a total thickness of 0.7 mm, which could require increased tooth reduction.

Declining Fortunes of Two Maxillary Incisors

4

Ceramics by Eva Forst, Newbury, UK

Pre- and Postoperative Status

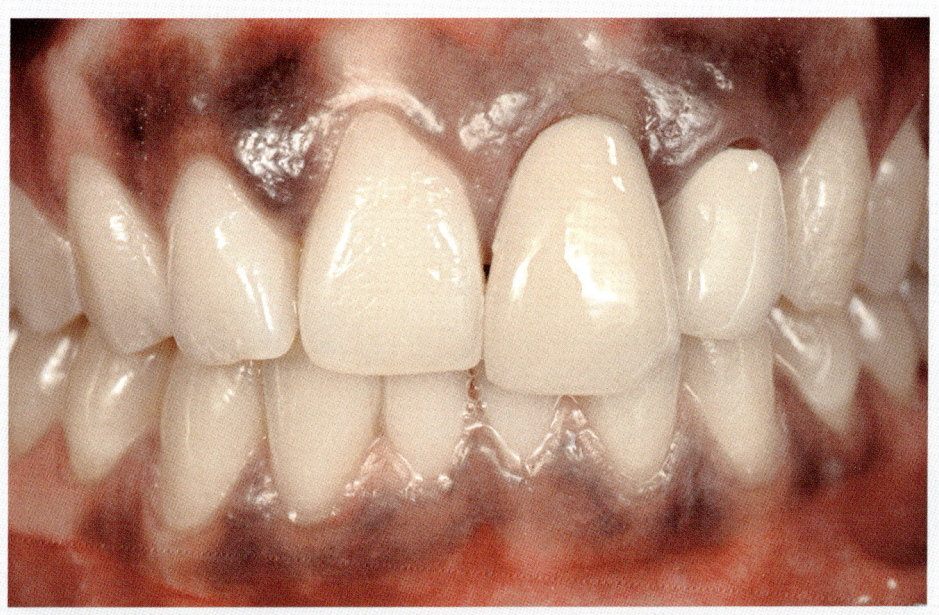

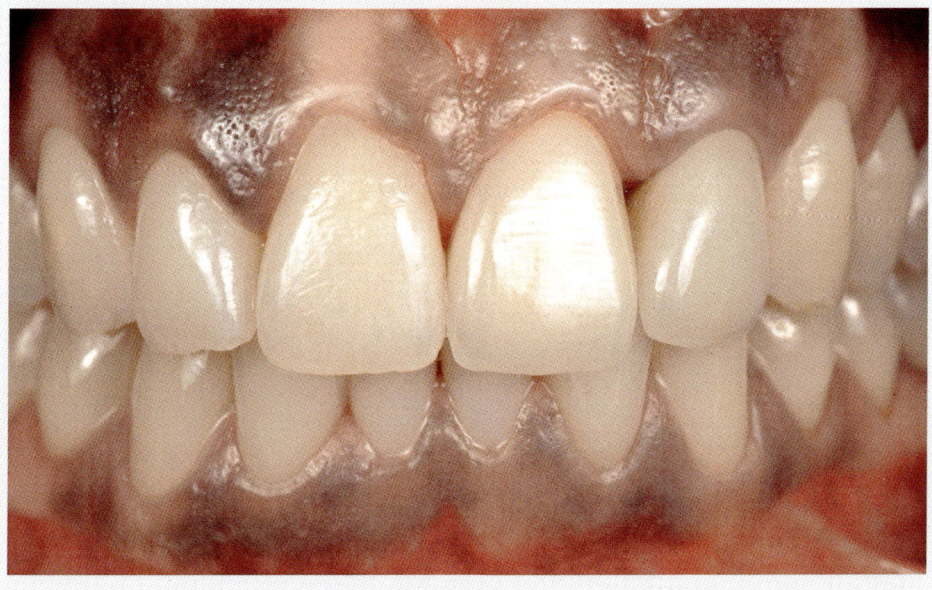

4 Declining Fortunes of Two Maxillary Incisors

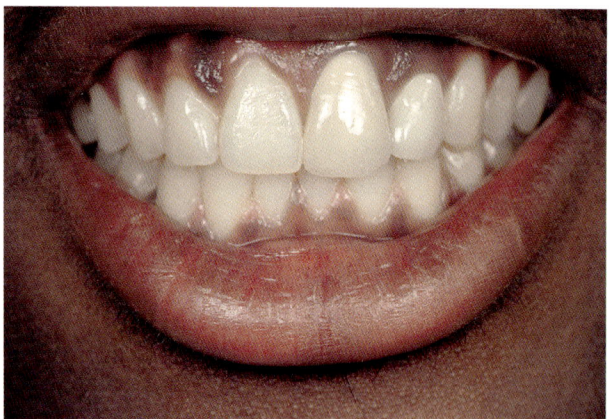

Fig 4-1 Dento-facial view: 2000.

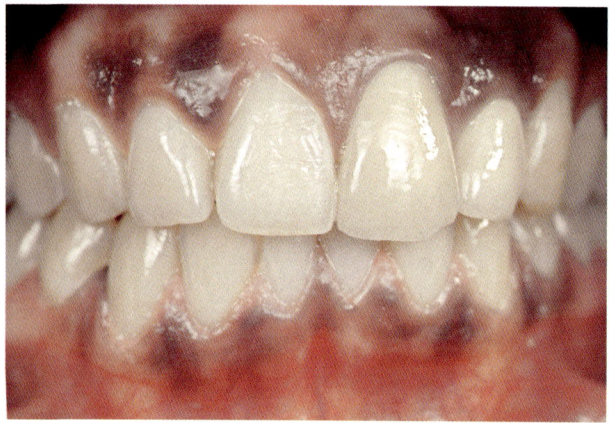

Fig 4-2 Anterior view in centric occlusion: 2000.

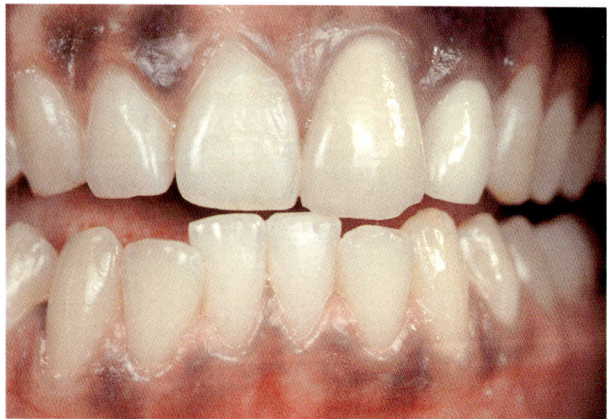

Fig 4-3 Anterior view in protrusive excursion: 2000.

Dental History

In 1996, at the age of 14 years, the patient was involved in a road traffic accident, which traumatized and devitalized his maxillary left central and lateral incisors. The lateral was mobile and the central avulsed. Both teeth were splinted for 6 weeks for stability and to allow undisturbed healing. Subsequently, periapical lesions developed on both teeth, necessitating root canal therapy. To mask the ensuing discoloration of the teeth and the metal posts and cores, two full-coverage metal-ceramic crowns were provided in 1997. Three years later in 2000, the patient attended with a distal porcelain fracture of the crown on the left central incisor (Fig 4-1).

Preoperative Status

The crown on the left central incisor lacked radiating symmetry, with a high gloss texture and luster compared with the natural right central incisor. In addition, the gingival zenith of the right central incisor undulated, peaking distally to the long axis of the tooth. This was dissimilar to the free gingival margin (FGM) around the crown on the left central incisor (Figs 4-2 to 4-4).

The cause of the porcelain fracture was interferences from the buccally placed mandibular left lateral incisor and canine, with insufficient occlusal clearance to accommodate the thickness of metal and porcelain of the crowns on maxillary left central and lateral incisors. The patient was referred for an orthodontic consultation to assess the feasibility of realigning the mandibular arch, which would eliminate the imbrications and create the requisite occlusal clearance for restorative materials. However, because the patient was studying at a university remote from home, he failed to follow up the orthodontic appointment.

In 2004, after completing university, the patient attended the practice, complaining of extrusion of the maxillary left central incisor, with a further porcelain fracture of the crown on the left lateral incisor (Figs 4-5 to 4-11). Examination and history taking

4 Declining Fortunes of Two Maxillary Incisors

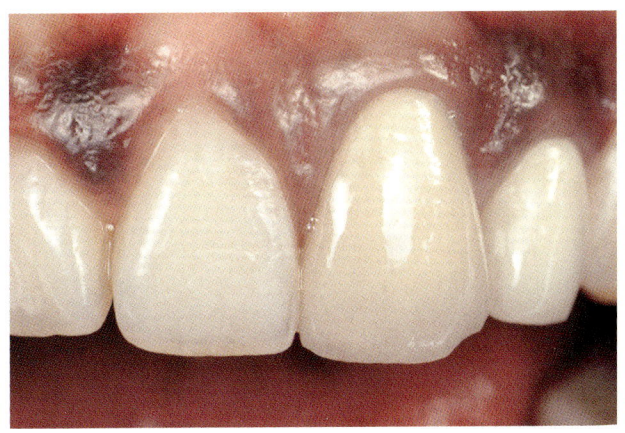

Fig 4-4 Anterior view showing fractured porcelain of metal-ceramic crown on left central incisor: 2000.

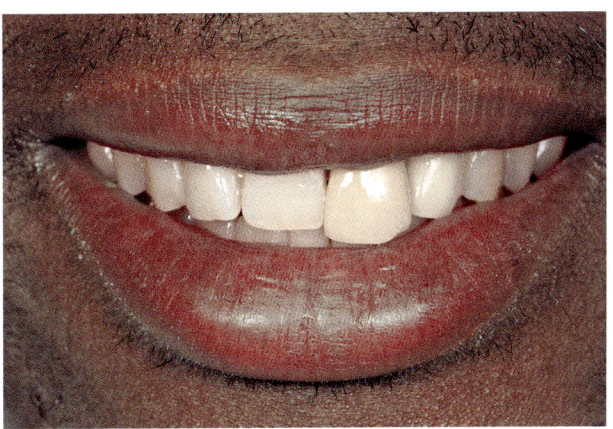

Fig 4-5 Dento-facial view: 2004.

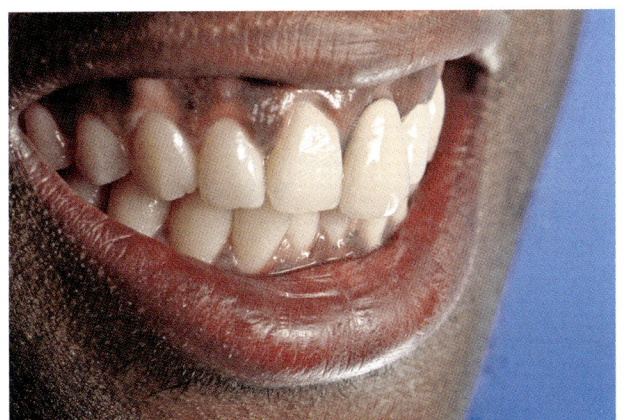

Fig 4-6 Right lateral dento-facial view in centric occlusion: 2004.

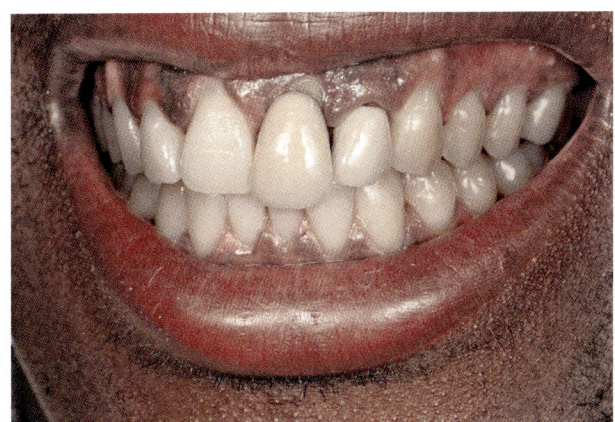

Fig 4-7 Left lateral dento-facial view in centric occlusion: 2004.

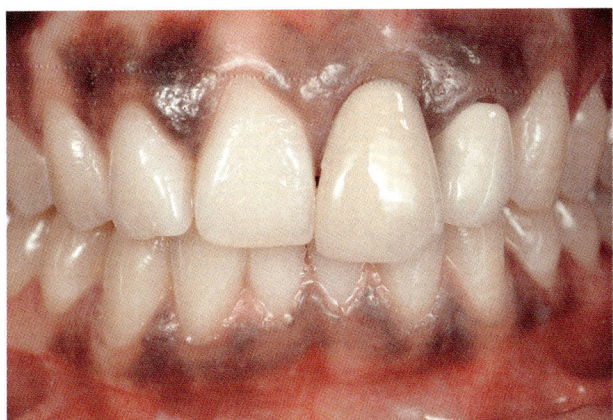

Fig 4-8 Anterior view in centric occlusion: 2004

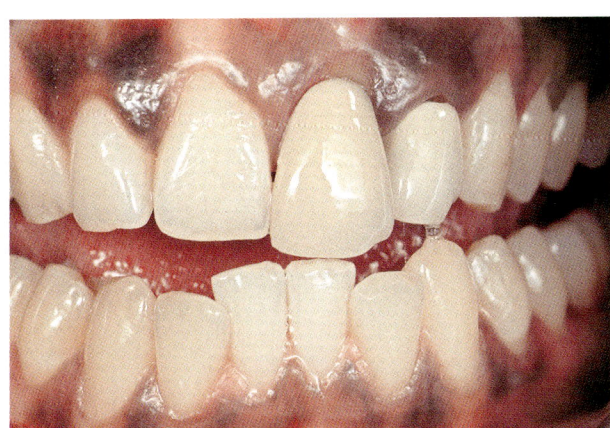

Fig 4-9 Anterior view in protrusive excursion: 2004.

4 Declining Fortunes of Two Maxillary Incisors

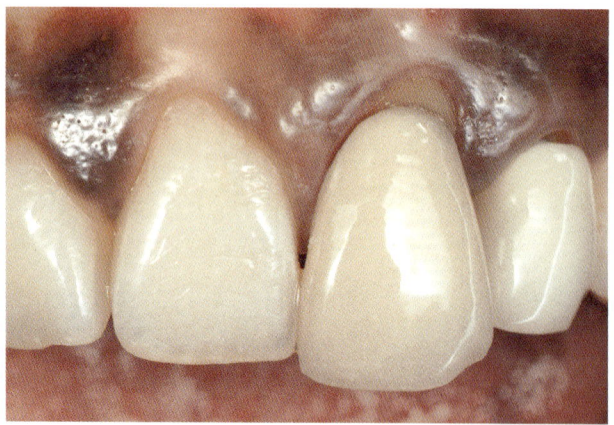

Fig 4-10 Anterior view showing fractured porcelain of metal-ceramic crowns on left central and lateral incisors and extrusion of left central incisors: 2004.

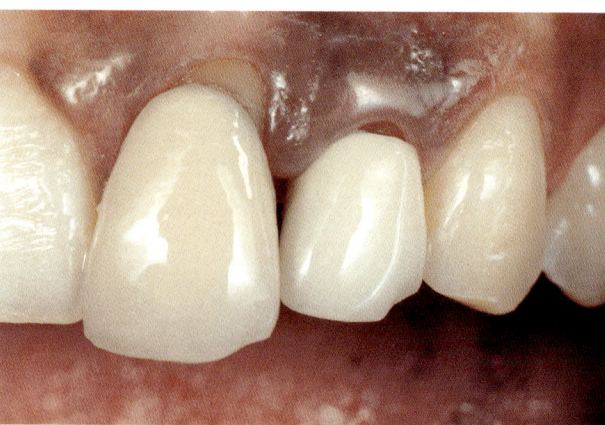

Fig 4-11 Left lateral view showing fractured porcelain of metal-ceramic crowns on left central and lateral incisors: 2004.

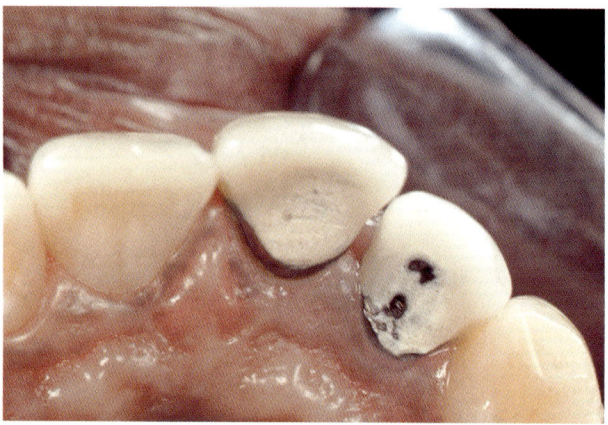

Fig 4-12 Incisal view showing occlusion adjustment of metal-ceramic crown on left lateral incisor: 2004.

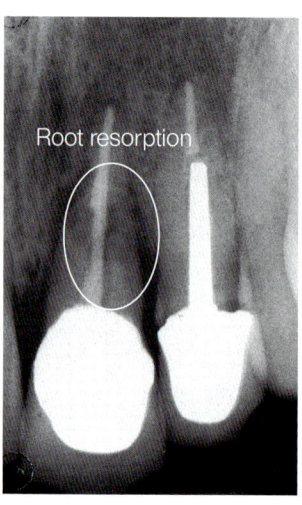

Fig 4-13 Radiograph showing radiolucency and root resorption related to left central incisor: 2004.

revealed that the university's dentist had adjusted the occlusion by grinding the palatal porcelain on both crowns (Fig 4-12). A periapical radiograph shows defective crown margins, periapical lesions, and root resorption related to the central incisor (Fig 4-13).

Treatment Options

1. Orthodontic realignment of the lower arch to gain space for restorative materials, and therefore prevent the mandibular left lateral incisor and canine grinding, as preparation for subsequent treatment options (Fig 4-14).
2. Extract the left central incisor and replace with a removable acrylic-resin partial denture and a new crown on the left lateral incisor (Fig 4-15).

4 Declining Fortunes of Two Maxillary Incisors

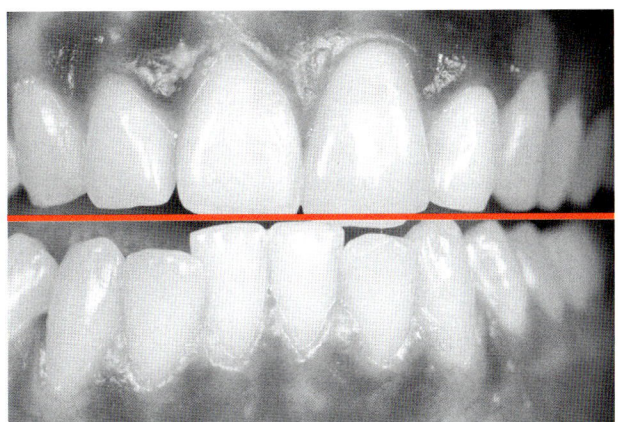

Fig 4-14 Option 1: orthodontic realignment of the lower arch, as preparation for subsequent treatment options.

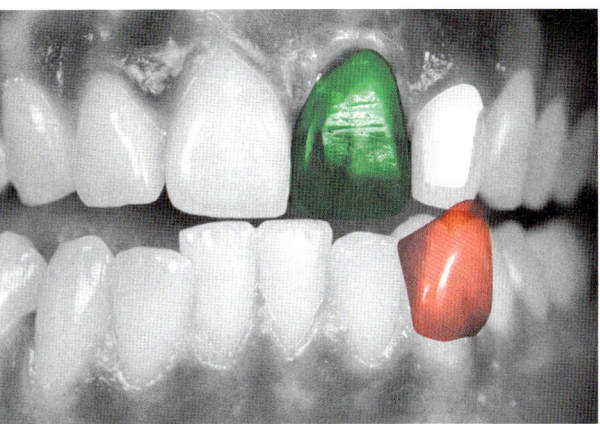

Fig 4-15 Option 2: removable acrylic-resin partial denture (green) and a new crown (red) on the left lateral incisor.

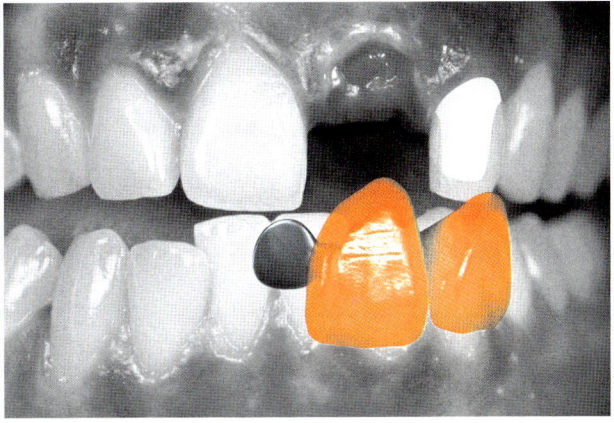

Fig 4-16 Option 3: two-unit cantilever bridge (orange) using the left lateral as an abutment tooth and a palatal wing on the right central incisor.

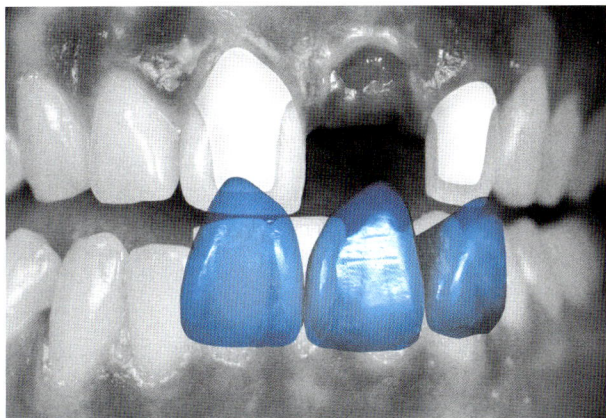

Fig 4-17 Option 4: three-unit fixed partial denture (blue), using the right central and left lateral incisors as abutments.

3. Extract the left central incisor and replace with a two-unit cantilever bridge using the left lateral as an abutment and a palatal wing on the right central incisor (Fig 4-16).
4. Extract the left central incisor and replace with a three-unit fixed partial denture, using the right central and left lateral incisors as abutments (Fig 4-17).
5. Extract the left central incisor and replace with an implant-supported crown, and place a new crown on the left lateral incisor (Fig 4-18).

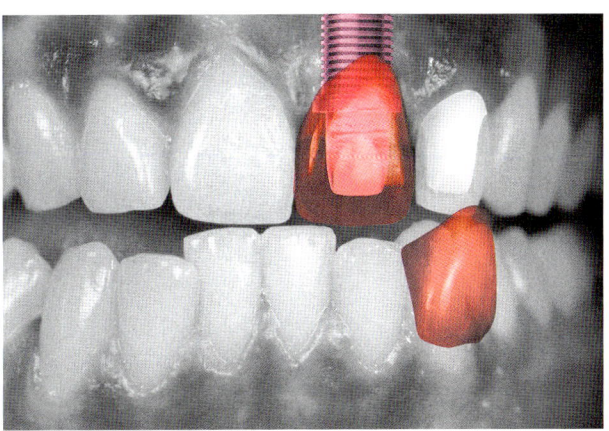

Fig 4-18 Option 5: implant-supported crown (red), and a new crown on the left lateral incisor.

Scientific Credence for Treatment Options

Realigning the lower arch would be minimally invasive and achieve the objectives of eliminating imbrications and creating the desired space for restorative materials. However, the therapy is protracted and, to prevent relapse, requires retention with either a removable appliance (with possible poor compliance) or a fixed lingual wire on the mandibular anterior teeth.

There is little doubt that the central incisor has poor prognosis and requires extraction. Replacement with a partial denture is economical, but it would be a social embarrassment as the patient is young and socially active. Furthermore, future recession at the extraction site would cause dislodgement, requiring future re-lining or replacement of the acyclic-resin prosthesis. A cantilever bridge would also be susceptible to dislodgment, and frequent recementing is onerous. Furthermore, recession at the extraction site is a potential food trap. The fixed partial denture option is highly destructive, requiring tooth preparation of the healthy right central incisor. As with the last two options, future bone remodeling and gingival recession at the extraction sites are potential problems. Finally, the implant option is feasible, but owing to the prevailing periapical lesion, the site is compromised by reduced vascularity, which can retard healing and osseointegration. In addition, extraction without augmentation or orthodontic extrusion could severely compromise soft tissue appearance at this esthetically sensitive region of the mouth.

Clinical Erudition and Feasibility

The provision of removable or fixed prostheses is within the remit of the practitioner. The implant option, however, is not as easy as it appears. The challenges are as follows:
- strategically timed extraction of the left central incisor, after orthodontic extrusion, to move the dento-gingival complex apically and prevent further bone loss
- review soft and hard tissue augmentation if the orthodontic route does not yield sufficient tissue volume
- sculpt the gingival contour around the implant with an accurate and correctly contoured provisional crown, so that the FGM mimics the unique undulations and peaks of the natural right central incisor
- two-stage surgery to allow revascularization of the site compromised by the periapical endodontic lesion
- employ a skilled ceramicist to fabricate both provisional and definitive crowns.

Patient Needs and Wants

A partial denture was unacceptable, and the patient desired a fixed option for his dental predicament. Although the patient accepted orthodontic treatment to extrude the maxillary right central incisor, he did not like the idea of wearing a removable retainer or having a fixed one on his lower teeth. He was therefore willing to accept grinding of the mandibular left lateral and canine, with the knowledge of the drawbacks of this procedure.

The first fixed option, the cantilever bridge, was declined on the grounds of instability. Tooth preparation for the three-unit fixed partial denture was refused based on the extensive damage required to a healthy natural tooth (right central incisor).

Although the implant option would be both protracted and costly, it has the advantages of a fixed option but without involving the adjacent teeth. This is the option that the patient agreed to proceed with, having being informed about the "pros and cons" of this treatment plan.

Treatment Sequence

The treatment started in September 2004 with the removal of the defective bonded crown on the left lateral incisor and its replacement with a chairside-fabricated acrylic-resin provisional crown. Shortly afterwards, orthodontic brackets were placed to extrude the left central incisor rapidly (Figs 4-19 to 4-21). The orthodontic appliances were periodically adjusted as periodontal growth proceeded, moving the entire dento-gingival complex coronally. During the following 8 months, the occlusion was also adjusted to compensate for coronal movement (Fig 4-22). Comparisons of radiographs taken in September 2004 and May 2005 clearly show coronal migration of the root and bone of the left central incisor (Figs 4-23 and 4-24).

A few weeks later, in June, 2005, a full-thickness flap was raised and the left central incisor extracted without traumatizing the buccal bone plate. Concurrently, curettage of the area was performed and the site augmented with Bio-Oss (Geistlich, UK) (Fig 4-25). A prefabricated provisional cantilever bridge, using the left lateral incisor as an abutment and a palatal wing on the right central incisor, was fitted immediately after suturing. A healing period of 12 months (which was longer than usual) was allowed to encourage vascularization and expedite osseointegration before the fixture was placed. During this healing phase, the cantilever bridge, which was not esthetically ideal, frequently dislodged and was occlusally adjusted and periodically recemented (Figs 4-26 to 4-29).

After 1 year, the site at the left central incisor was overaugmented. This overcompensation by grafting is advantageous and a precaution for postoperative recession after implant placement (Figs 4-30 and 4-31). In April 2006, a Tapered Groovy RP 4.3 mm × 13 mm implant (Nobel Biocare, Sweden) was placed via a palatal peninsular flap. This type of palatal flap reduces trauma and minimizes buccal recession and scarring to a site that has already undergone augmentation from the buccal aspect (Figs 4-32 and 4-33). After placing the fixture and suturing, the temporary cantilever bridge was recemented.

4 Declining Fortunes of Two Maxillary Incisors

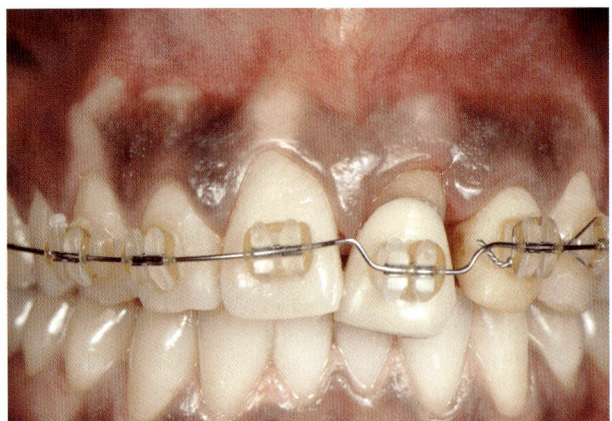

Fig 4-19 Orthodontic extrusion of left central incisor: centric occlusion.

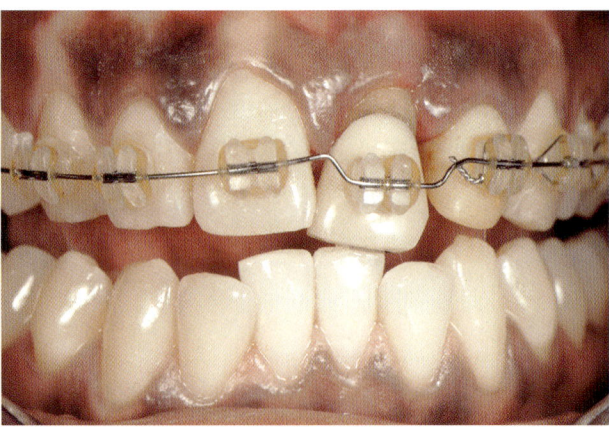

Fig 4-20 Orthodontic extrusion of left central incisor: protrusion.

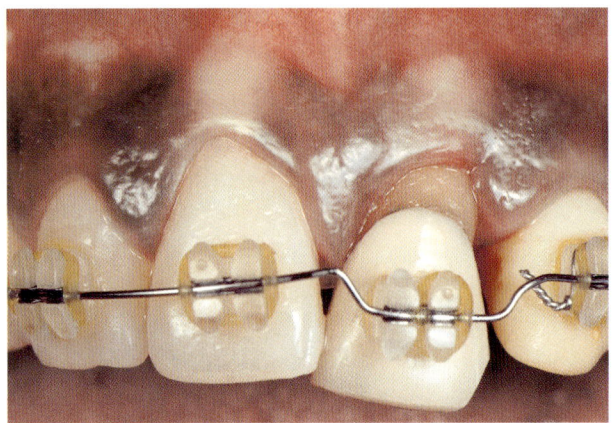

Fig 4-21 Orthodontic extrusion of left central incisor: notice acrylic-resin provisional crown on left lateral incisor.

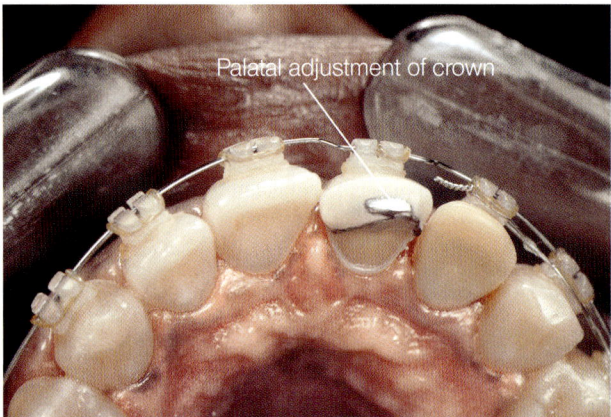

Fig 4-22 Orthodontic extrusion of left central incisor: incisal view.

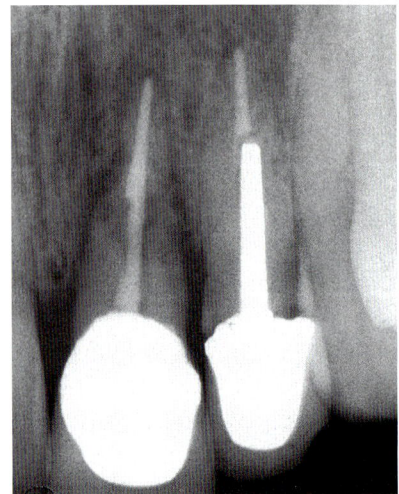

Fig 4-23 Radiograph: September 2004.

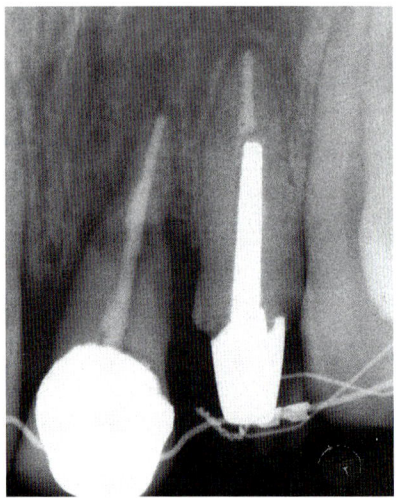

Fig 4-24 Radiograph: May 2005.

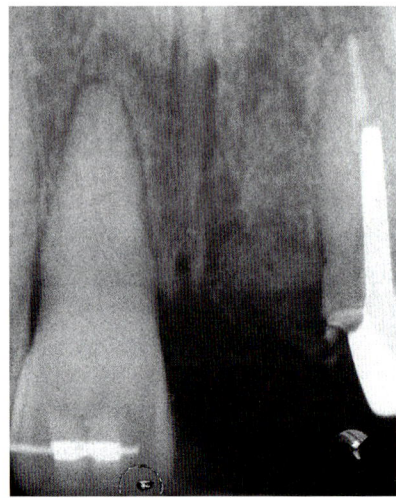

Fig 4-25 Radiograph following extraction of left central incisor and bone grafting: June 2005.

4 Declining Fortunes of Two Maxillary Incisors

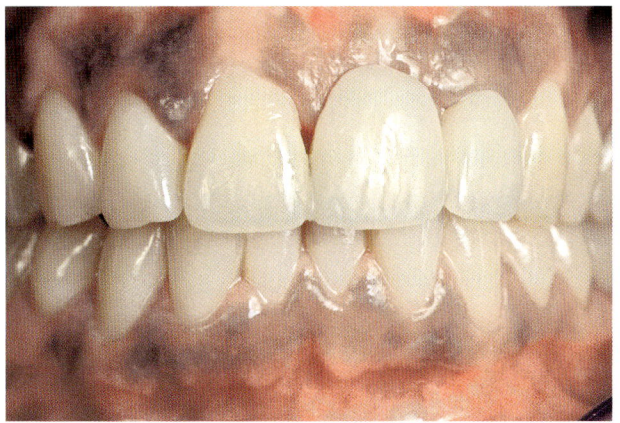

Fig 4-26 Provisional cantilever bridge: centric occlusion.

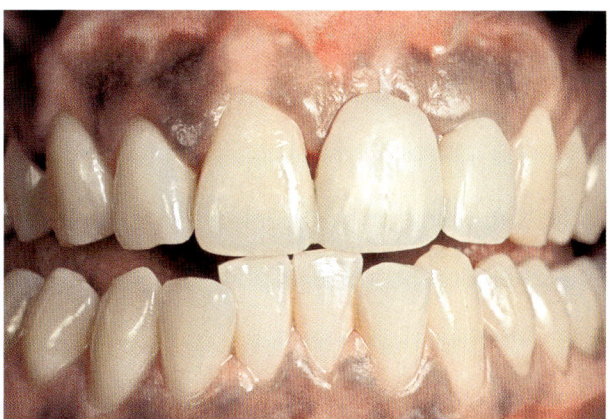

Fig 4-27 Provisional cantilever bridge: protrusion.

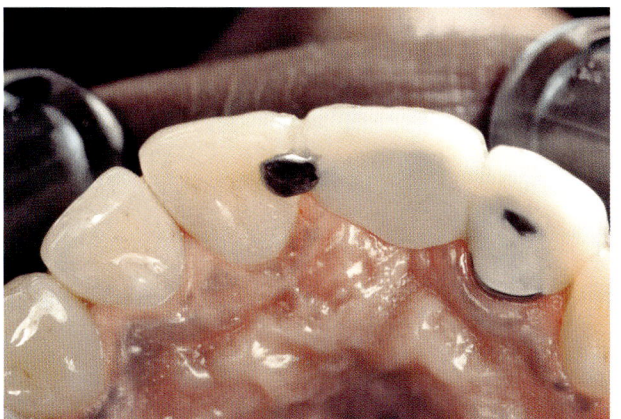

Fig 4-28 Provisional cantilever bridge: incisal view.

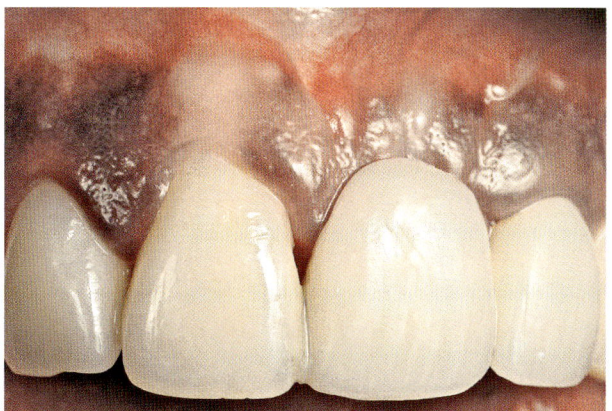

Fig 4-29 Provisional cantilever bridge: anterior view.

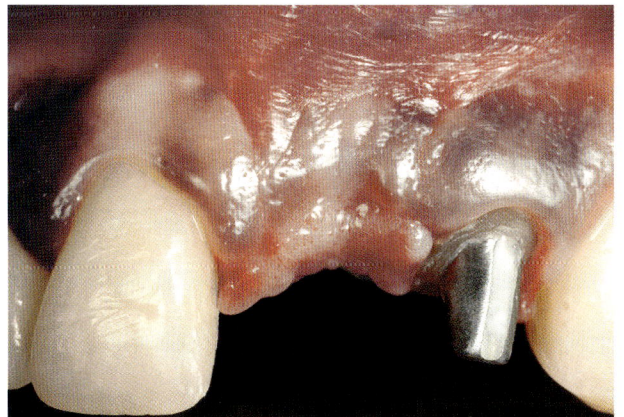

Fig 4-30 Healed left central incisor site: anterior view.

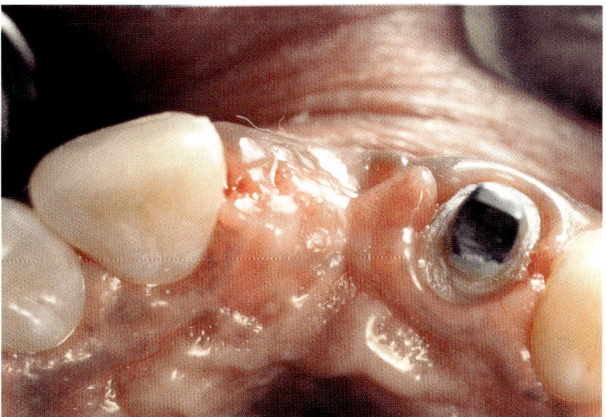

Fig 4-31 Healed left central incisor site: incisal view.

4 Declining Fortunes of Two Maxillary Incisors

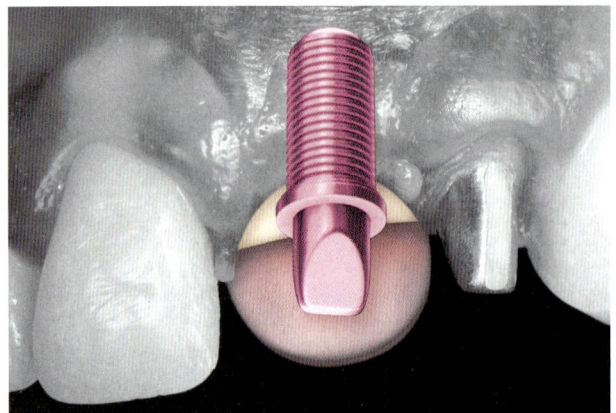

Fig 4-32 Palatal peninsular flap for placement of the implant: anterior view. The flap is peeled away, revealing the bone underneath, allowing placement of the implant.

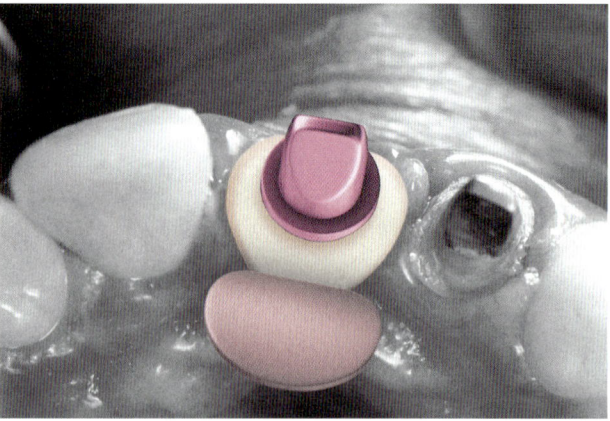

Fig 4-33 Palatal peninsular flap for placement of the implant: incisal view.

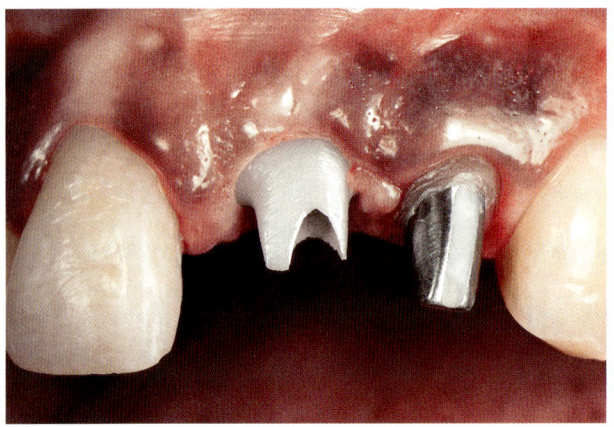

Fig 4-34 Zirconia abutment: anterior view.

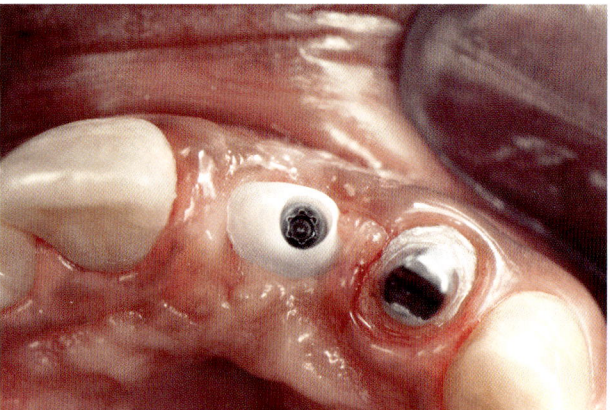

Fig 4-35 Zirconia abutment: incisal view.

After 6 months, in October 2006, a tissue punch was used to expose the implant and a fixture level impression was made to fabricate a custom zirconia abutment. A healing cap was placed in the interim while awaiting the zirconia abutment. Upon delivery from the dental laboratory, the zirconia abutment was screwed onto the fixture, but its cervico-incisal length was short, resulting in poor retention and causing frequent dislodgment of the provisional crown (Figs 4-34 and 4-35). Although the temporary crown on the left central incisor was shorter and wider than the natural right counterpart, it served its purpose by sculpting the FGM (Figs 4-36 to 4-39). In order to mimic the unique undulations and peaks of the FGM of the right central incisor, the temporary crown on the left central incisor was periodically adjusted as follows. To encourage coronal regrowth of the FGM (creep), the cervical region of the crown was contoured to attenuate

4 Declining Fortunes of Two Maxillary Incisors

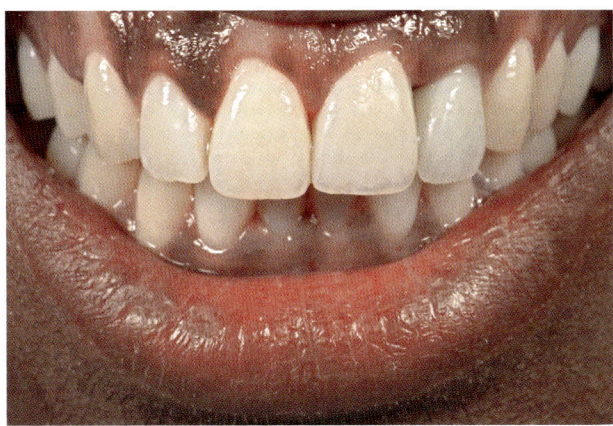

Fig 4-36 Provisional crowns on left central and lateral incisors: dento-facial view.

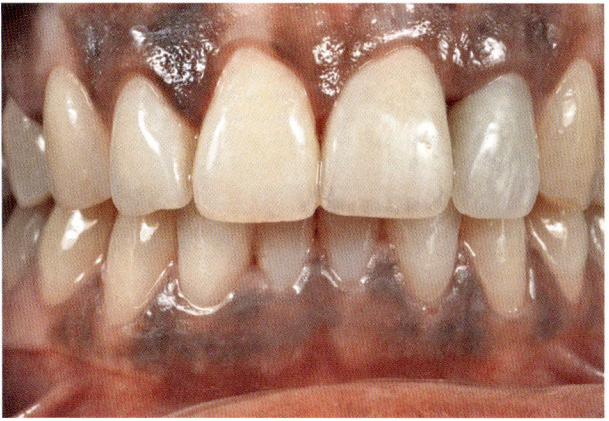

Fig 4-37 Provisional crowns on left central and lateral incisors: centric occlusion.

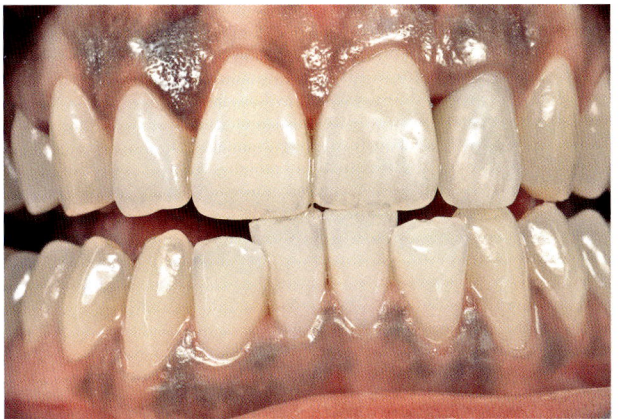

Fig 4-38 Provisional crowns on left central and lateral incisors: protrusion.

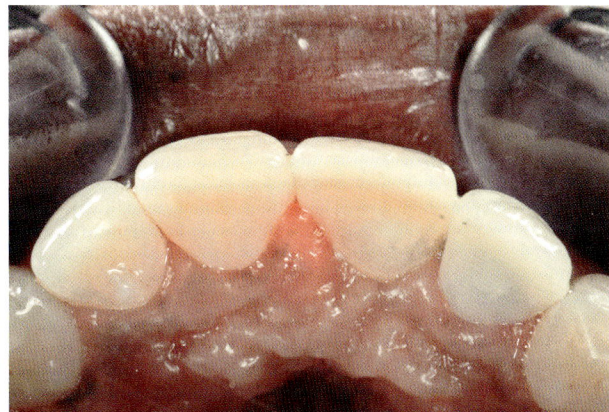

Fig 4-39 Provisional crowns on left central and lateral incisors: incisal view.

the convex acuity (flat or concave profile). The opposite was necessary for apical migration of the FGM (recession) that is, to accentuate convex acuity (convex profile) (Figs 4-40 and 4-41). The crowns also served the purpose of assessing occlusion and phonetics, and adjustments were made accordingly.

Four months later, in February 2007, impressions were made to transfer the contour of the transmucosal tissues to the laboratory for fabricating the definitive crowns with the correct emergence profiles. A new zirconia abutment was fabricated, which was longer and with improved retention (Fig 4-42). The abutments of the left central (zirconia) and lateral (metal core) incisors were scanned and, using computer-aided design and computer-assisted manufacture software, two Procera (Nobel Biocare, Sweden) crowns were fabricated with 0.4 mm alumina copings (Figs 4-43 and 4-44).

4 Declining Fortunes of Two Maxillary Incisors

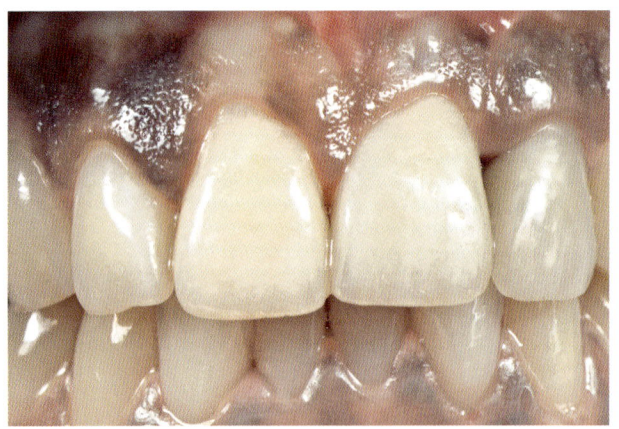

Fig 4-40 Provisional crowns on left central and lateral incisors: anterior view.

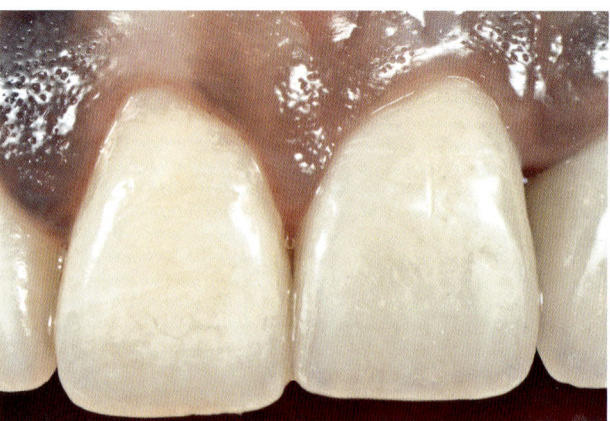

Fig 4-41 Provisional crowns on left central and lateral incisors: notice the sculptured FGM at the left central incisor site, mimicking that around the natural right central incisor.

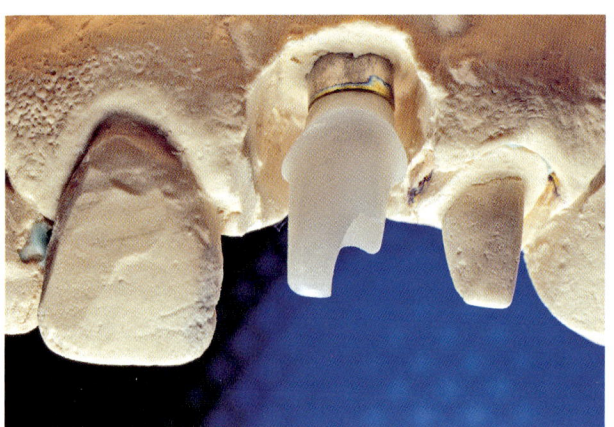

Fig 4-42 The second, longer zirconia abutment with improved retention.

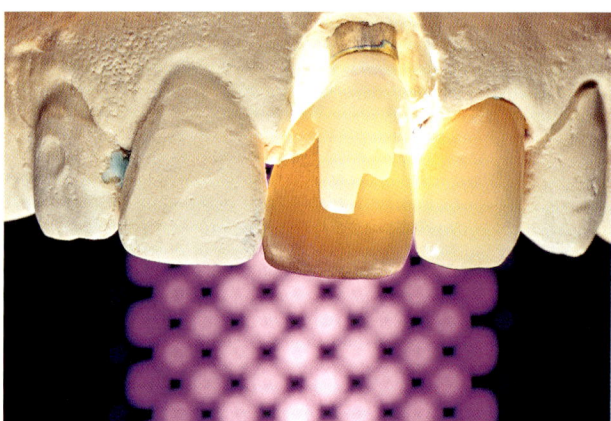

Fig 4-43 Procera crown being fabricated onto the zirconia abutment.

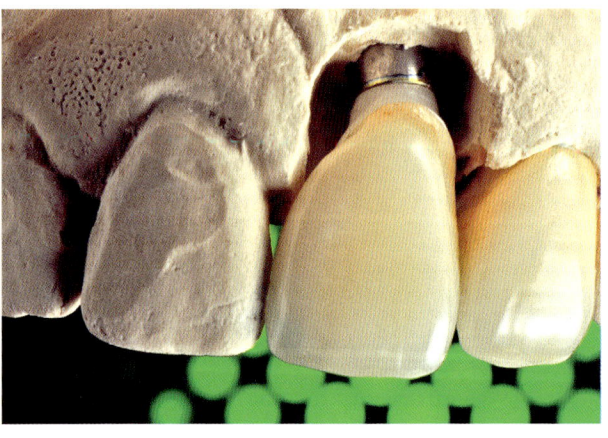

Fig 4-44 Completed Procera crowns for left central and lateral incisors.

4 Declining Fortunes of Two Maxillary Incisors

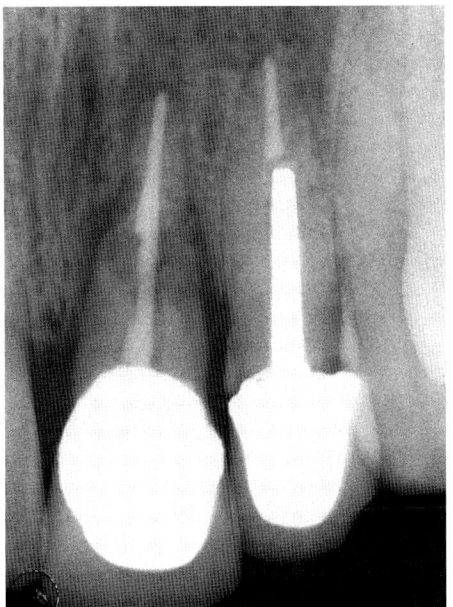

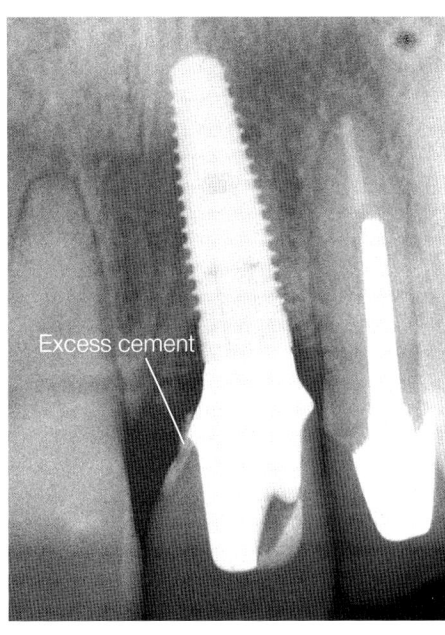

Fig 4-45 Radiograph: September 2004.

Fig 4-46 Radiograph: March 2007.

Preoperative (September 2004) and postoperative (March 2007) radiographs (Figs 4-45 and 4-46) show correctly fitting crowns with successful integration of the implant at the left central incisor site. Notice the excess cement mesial to the crown on the implant, which was subsequently removed.

Pre- and postoperative sequences are shown in Figs 4-47 to 4-58. A detailed analysis revealed the following (Fig 4-49):

- almost identical tissue scallop around the implant-supported crown at the left central site, mimicking the undulations and peaks of the FGM around the natural right central incisor
- presence of a median interdental papilla
- impeccable integration of the crowns with the adjacent and antagonist natural dentition.

Discussion

Comparisons of the pre- and postoperative images show that the treatment objectives – to resolve anterior dental esthetic anomalies – were achieved by providing fixed prostheses. However, the sacrifice was that the mandibular left lateral incisor and canines required grinding to accommodate the restorative materials of the opposing crowns (Fig 4-54). In addition, scarring is evident on the attached gingivae, apical to the left central incisor, as a relic of the initial incisions when the tooth was extracted and the site augmented. Scarring is usually more pronounced with thick biotypes, but is almost inconsequential to dental esthetics in this case study, especially because of racial pigmentation of the gingivae, which camouflages the "defect". If desired, the scarring could be resolved by either scraping with a scalpel or using a soft-tissue laser.

4 Declining Fortunes of Two Maxillary Incisors

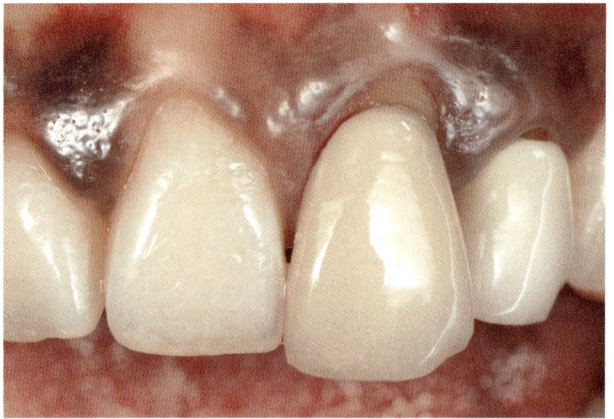

Fig 4-47 Preoperative anterior view: 2004.

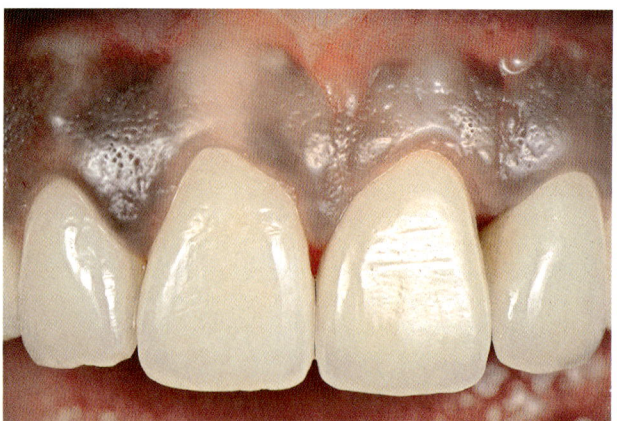

Fig 4-48 Postoperative anterior view: 2007.

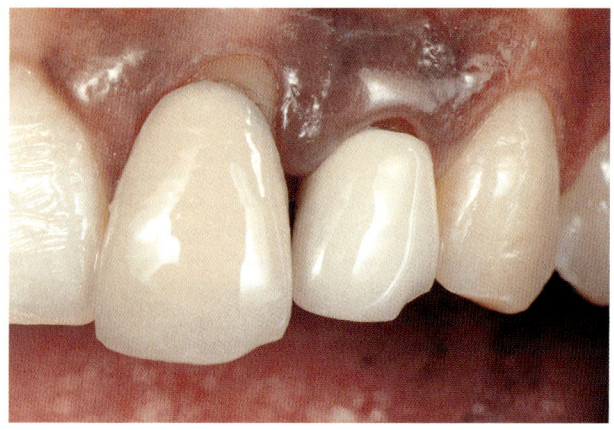

Fig 4-49 Preoperative left lateral view: 2004.

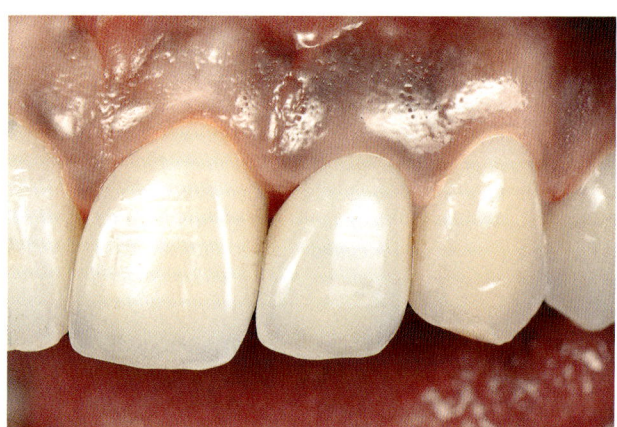

Fig 4-50 Postoperative left lateral view: 2007.

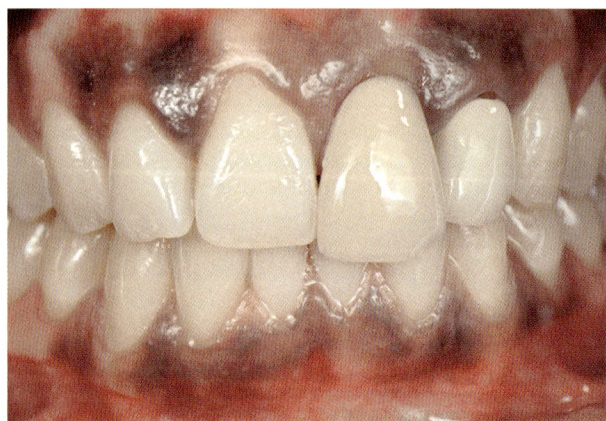

Fig 4-51 Preoperative centric occlusion: 2004.

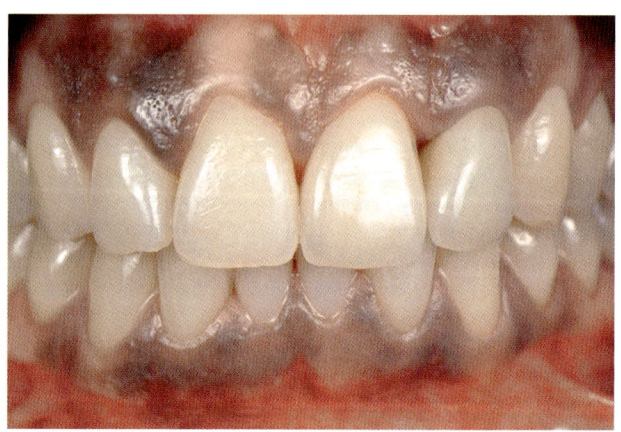

Fig 4-52 Postoperative centric occlusion: 2007.

4 Declining Fortunes of Two Maxillary Incisors

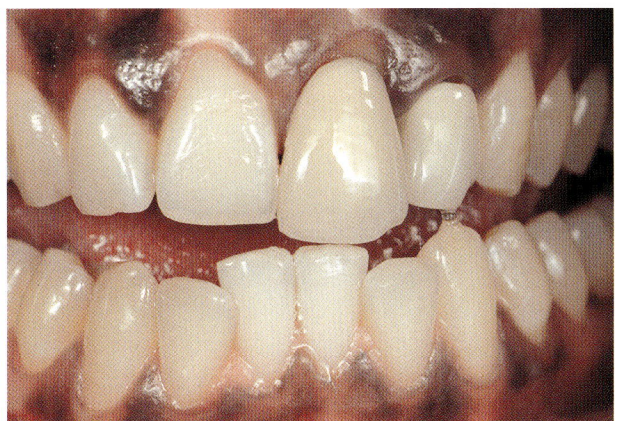

Fig 4-53 Preoperative protrusion: 2004.

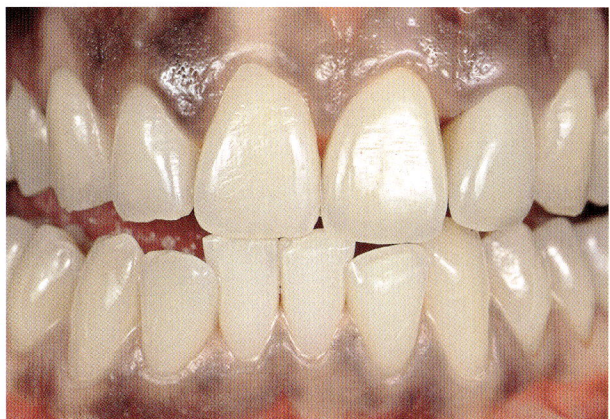

Fig 4-54 Postoperative protrusion: 2007.

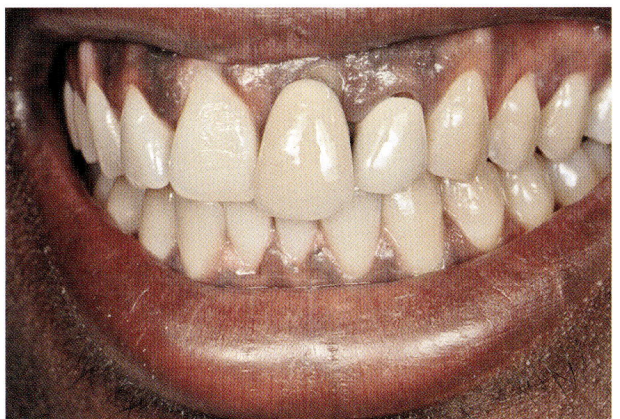

Fig 4-55 Preoperative dento-facial view: 2004.

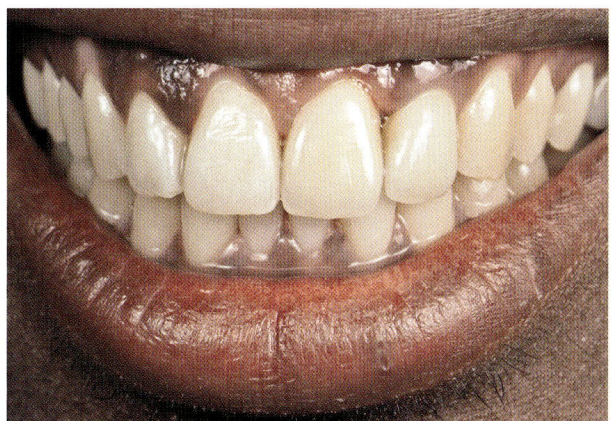

Fig 4-56 Postoperative dento-facial view: 2007.

It was unfortunate that the initial zirconia abutment was short and had to be replaced with a longer one. This protocol is far from ideal, because removing abutments and making impressions disrupts any epithelial or connective tissue attachments on the abutment from the transmucosal tissues. Another factor to mention is that the occlusion requires periodic monitoring to ensure that the crowns or the underlying implant abutment do not become loose. Finally, the treatment was protracted, taking nearly 2½ years to complete.

4 Declining Fortunes of Two Maxillary Incisors

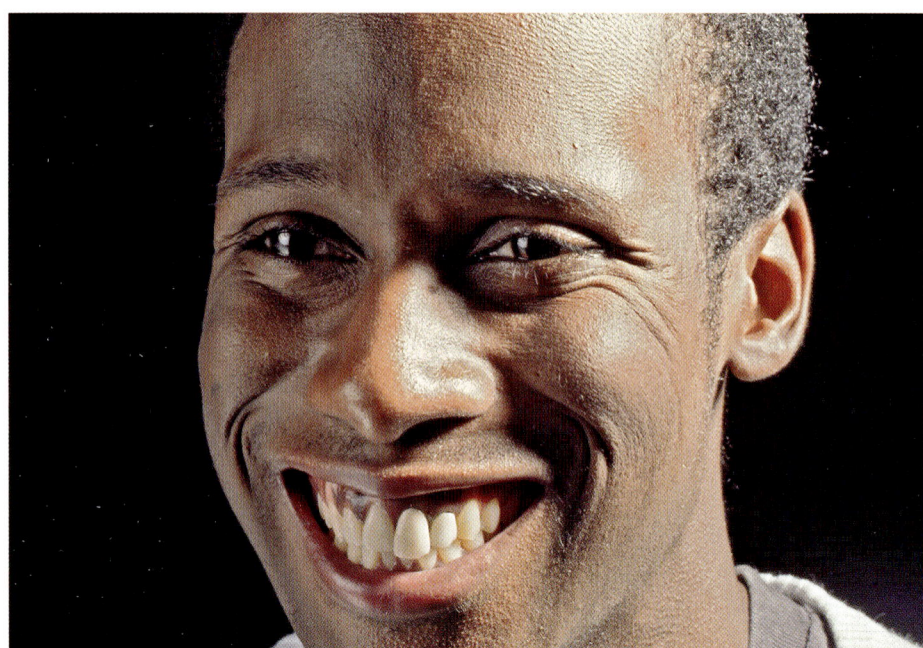

Fig 4-57 Preoperative facial view: 2004.

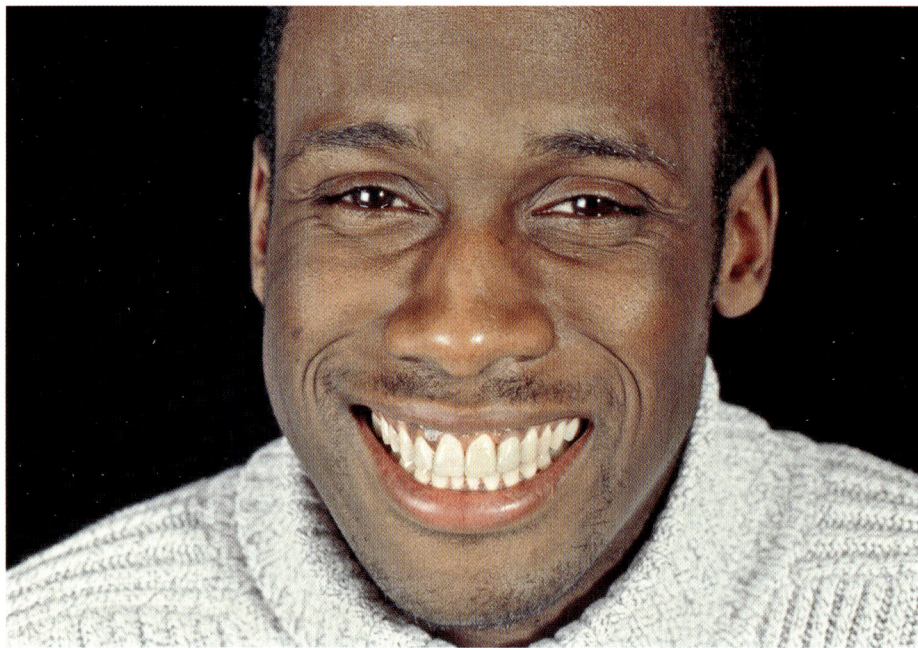

Fig 4-58 Postoperative facial view: 2007.

Traumatic Loss of Maxillary Central Incisors

Ceramics by Gérald Ubassy, Avignon, France

Pre- and Postoperative Status

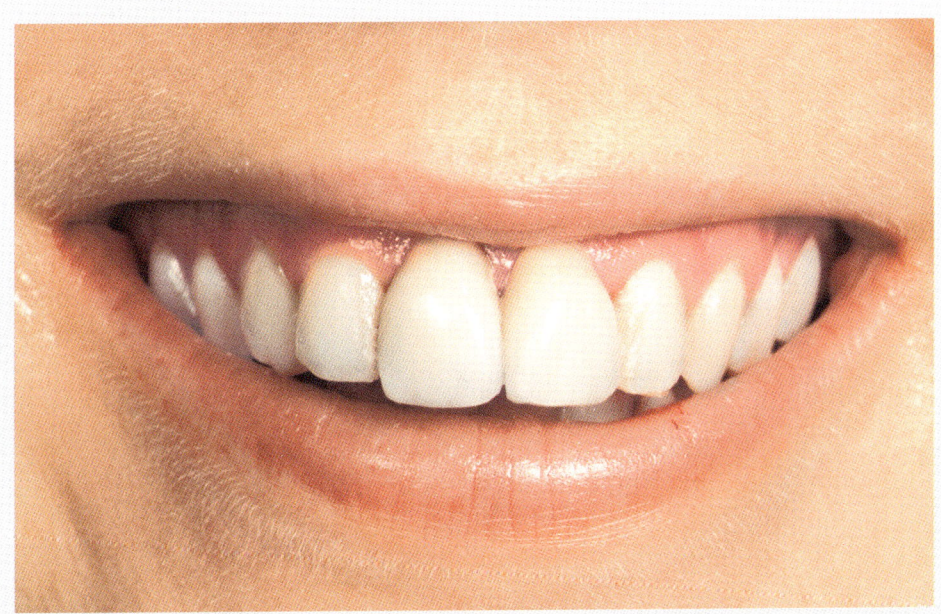

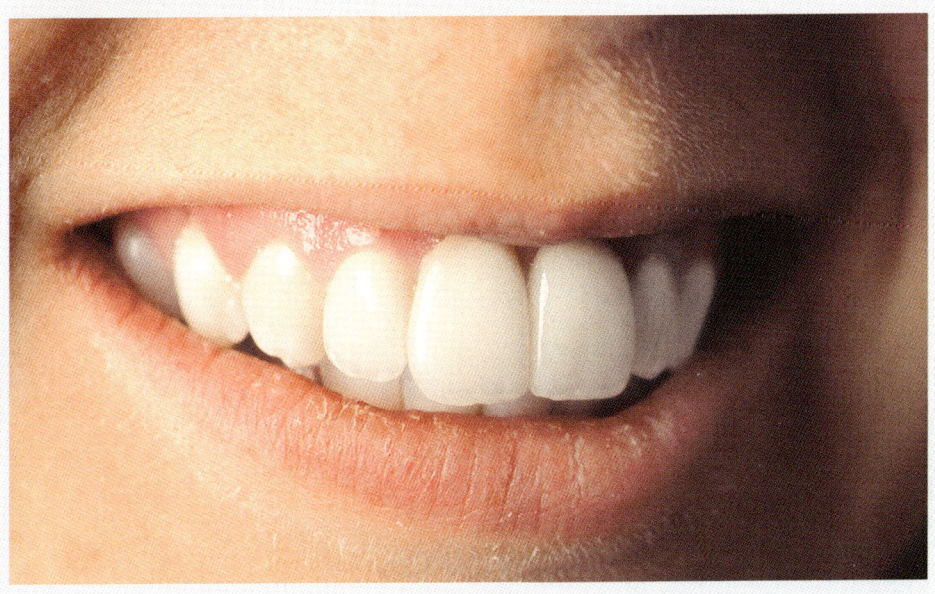

5 Traumatic Loss of Maxillary Central Incisors

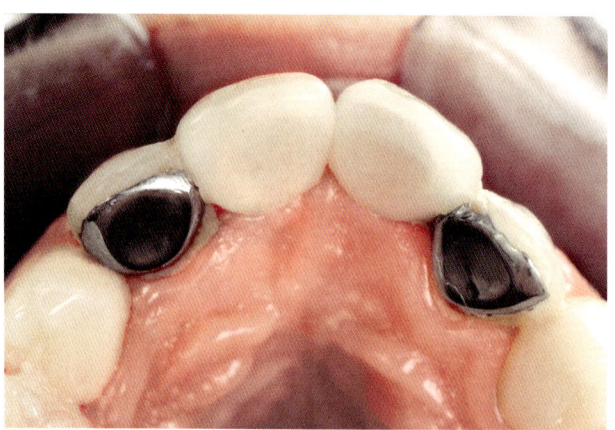

Fig 5-1 Preoperative view of two Rochette bridges replacing missing central incisors: incisal view.

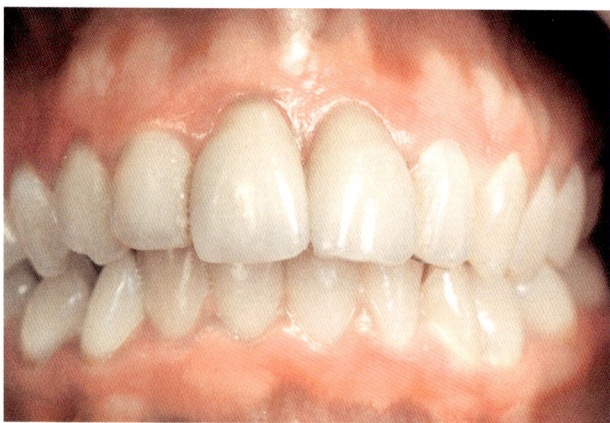

Fig 5-2 Preoperative view of two Rochette bridges replacing missing central incisors: anterior view.

Dental History

During her early teens, the patient lost her maxillary central incisors while diving into a swimming pool. After the trauma, she was provided with two Rochette bridges, which were unstable and perpetually dislodging. On one occasion, the bridges were lost and replacements provided, but with little improvement in stability. The patient yearned for a fixed prosthodontic solution, and at the age of 25 she decided to seek advice.

Preoperative Status

Extraoral examination revealed an average lip line, with the lower border of the upper lip touching the cervical aspect of the maxillary central incisors. The palatal wings of the two Rochette bridges on the lateral incisors were defective, encouraging plaque accumulation (Fig 5-1). The pontics replacing the missing central incisors were narrow and triangular shaped (Fig 5-2) compared with the patient's natural oval-shaped teeth prior to the accident (Fig 5-3). The ceramics were dire, with poor characterization, incorrect shape, and unsightly luster and texture. Excess cement was effusing at the mesial aspects of the laterals, adding to the cumulative effect of poor anterior esthetics.

The maxillary arch was narrow, terminating as a chevron at the central incisor region (Fig 5-4). In addition, the incisors were protruding with a vastly increased horizontal overjet of 7 mm (Figs 5-5 and 5-6). A periapical radiograph showed an open median maxillary fissure with mesially inclined roots of the lateral incisors (Fig 5-7).

5 Traumatic Loss of Maxillary Central Incisors

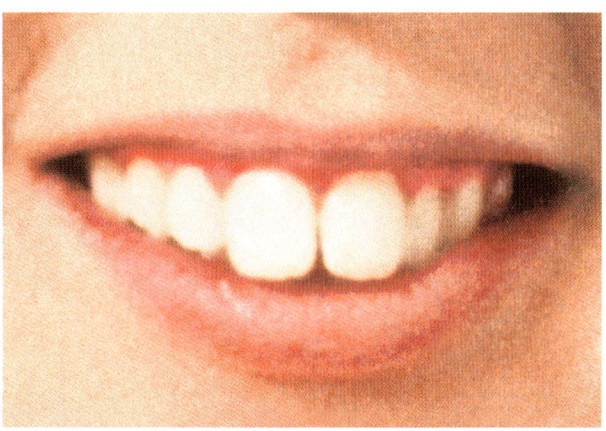

Fig 5-3 Natural central incisors prior to accident, during the patient's teens.

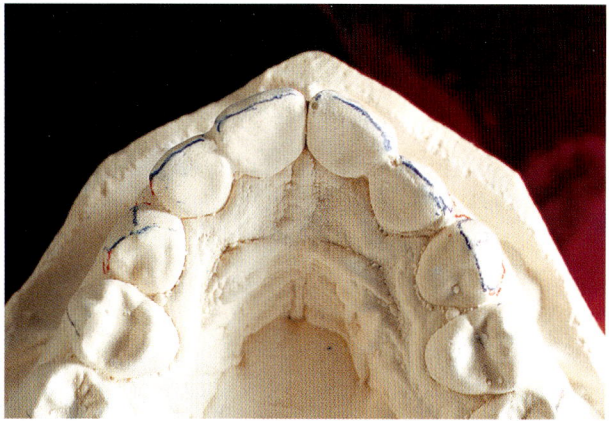

Fig 5-4 Plaster cast showing chevron-shaped maxillary arch.

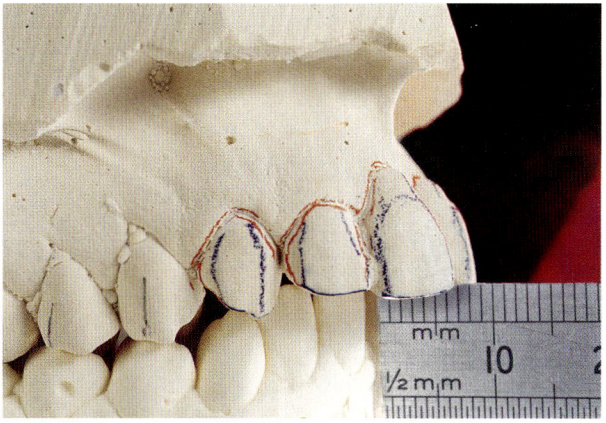

Fig 5-5 Right lateral view of plaster cast showing a horizontal overjet of 7 mm.

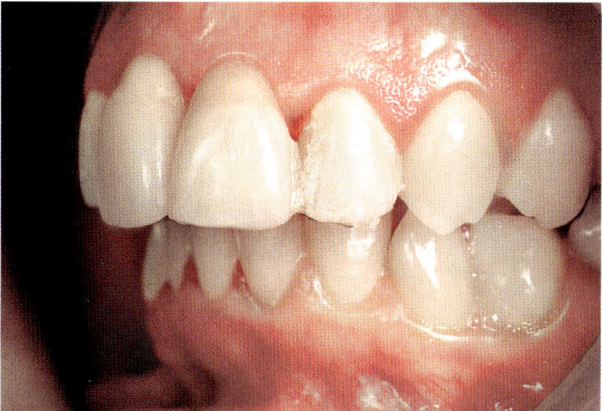

Fig 5-6 Left lateral view showing a pronounced horizontal overjet.

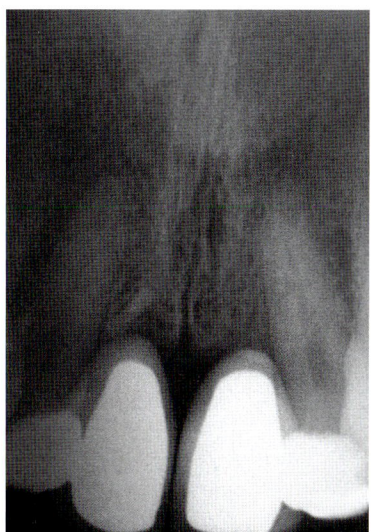

Fig 5-7 Preoperative radiograph showing Rochette bridges and mesial inclination of lateral incisor roots.

57

Treatment Options

1. Discard the Rochette bridges and provide a removable acrylic-resin partial denture (Fig 5-8).
2. One Rochette bridge or composite-resin fiber-reinforced fixed partial denture (FPD) with improved pontic esthetics (Fig 5-9).
3. Planned Le Forte fracture, followed by premaxilla retrusion to decrease the vast horizontal overjet, followed by prosthetic replacement of the central incisors by one of the other listed options (Fig 5-10).
4. Orthodontic treatment to distalize the mesially inclined roots of the lateral incisor, and convert the arch form to an oval shape, thereby creating space for placing two implant-supported crowns to replace the missing central incisors (Fig 5-11).
5. Four-unit FPD, using the two lateral incisors as abutments (Fig 5-12).

Scientific Credence for Treatment Options

The partial denture is the least invasive option but is predisposed to dislodgment, relining, and/or replacement. The orthognathic surgical option is obviously the most invasive and protracted, but it would achieve the objective of reducing the horizontal overjet. It would also be prophylactic by preventing undue trauma to the eventual prostheses replacing the missing central incisors. Orthodontic treatment is an alternative (possibly in conjunction with surgery) but would involve realignment of both arches, with permanent retention to prevent relapse. Both options 3 and 4 would potentially pave the way for implant-supported prostheses. The last option, an FPD, will be destructive, but offers better retention than a removable denture or a Rochette or fiber-reinforced bridge.

Clinical Erudition and Feasibility

The removable and fixed partial dentures are within the remit of the practitioner. However, experience and knowledge are required to sculpt the pontic sites to create an emergence profile that gives the pontics the appearance of emanating from the soft tissues – similar to natural teeth surrounded by a free gingival margin (FGM). Of course, employing a skilled ceramist is mandatory for creating life-like restorations.

For the remaining options (ie, surgery, orthodontics, and implants), specialist consultation or referral is advisable.

Patient Needs and Wants

The removable denture option was greeted with dismay, as was the thought of attempting another Rochette bridge. The latter choice was specifically dismissed based on the poor experience with the two previous similar prostheses.

5 Traumatic Loss of Maxillary Central Incisors

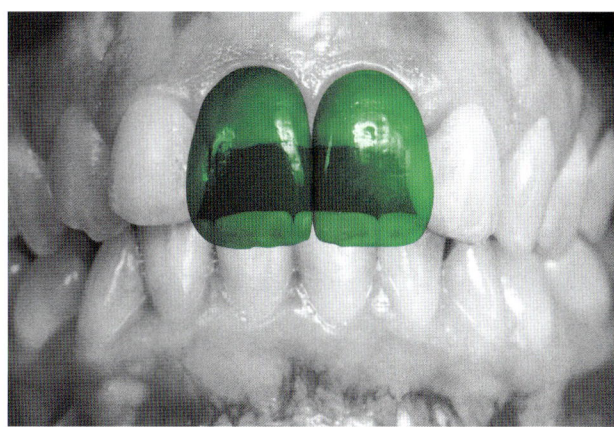

Fig 5-8 Option 1: acrylic-resin removable partial denture (green).

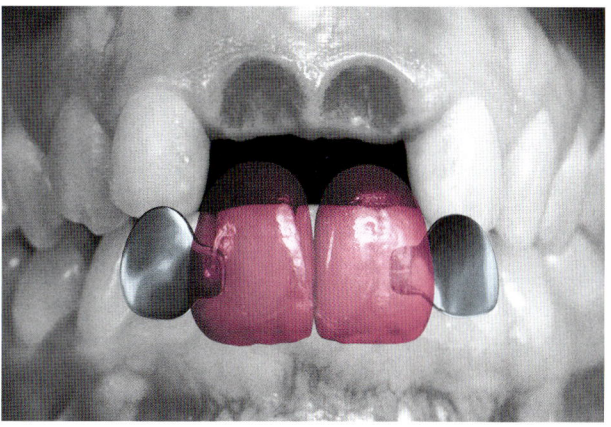

Fig 5-9 Option 2: Rochette bridge (purple), with palatal wings.

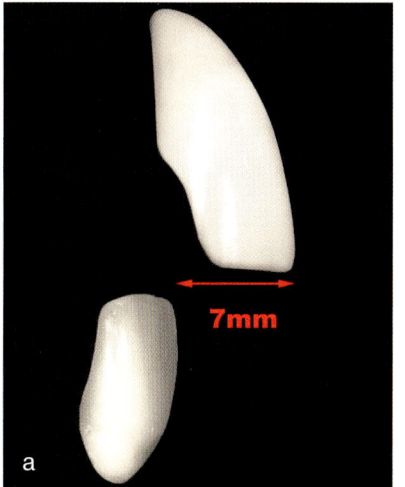
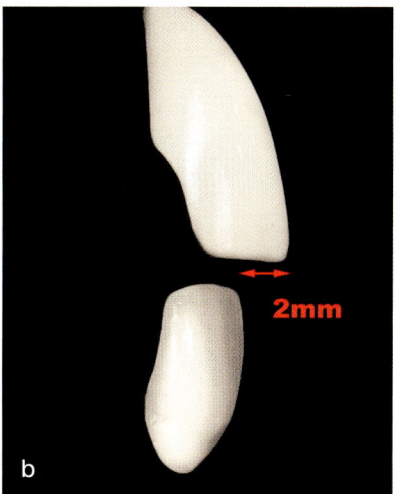

Fig 5-10a,b Option 3: Le Forte fracture followed by premaxilla retrusion to decrease the horizontal overjet.

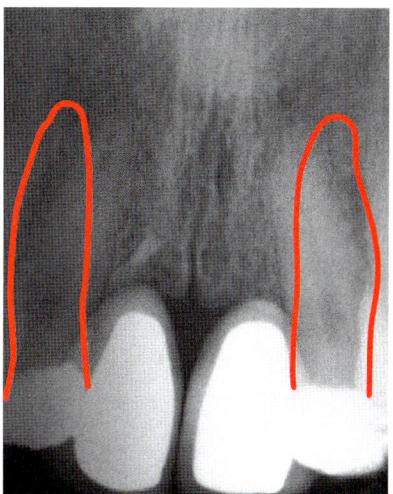

Fig 5-11 Option 4: orthodontic treatment to distalize the mesially inclined roots of the lateral incisors.

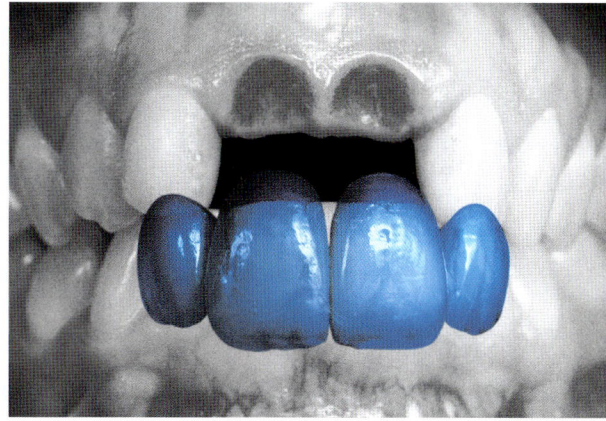

Fig 5-12 Option 5: four-unit fixed partial denture (blue), using the lateral incisors as abutments.

59

While the patient understood the long-term permanency of the surgical and orthodontic options, she refused both because of the lengthy treatment times. The only option remaining was that of an FPD, which would offer improved retention but would potentially sacrifice two vital, virgin teeth as abutments. The patient was informed about the possibility of future endodontic complications but chose to opt for this prosthodontic option.

Treatment Sequence

Having chosen the FPD option, the next decision was to choose between a metal-ceramic or all-ceramic prosthesis. A metal-ceramic prosthesis offers strength but lacks esthetics. This is particularly significant since the patient shows the cervical aspect of both lateral incisors during a relaxed smile and the cervical margins of the central incisor during an exaggerated smile.

Since esthetics were of paramount concern, ceramics were the better option. However, the weaker silica ceramics are unsuitable for FPDs, which leaves either the alumina or zirconia ceramics. In this instance, zirconia was chosen for its high strength, resilience at the connector sites, and its ability to withstand possible traumas from the vulnerable protrusive pontics. Although zirconia frameworks boast a flexural strength of over 1,000 MPa, the material has a low glass content, which means that light transmission is reduced compared with alumina and silica ceramics. The lack of translucency is challenging for creating natural, life-like restorations, and the ceramist often has to resort to complex porcelain layering techniques to overcome this optical drawback.

The initial stage was to draw line angles on the preoperative cast to visualize how to convert the triangular pontics to oval shapes (Fig 5-13). Next, the existing Rochette bridges were removed and the lateral incisors prepared by a 1.2 mm reduction and smooth shoulder margins. A chairside four-unit acrylic-resin FPD was fabricated with oval-shaped pontics. To sculpt the soft tissue, the cervical aspects were refined with concave apical rings to create pseudo FGMs, emulating those of the natural teeth. After 2 weeks of wearing the provisional partial denture, the sculptured pontic sites showed pseudo FGMs (Fig 5-14).

Once the tissue scallop was satisfactory, impressions were made and the plaster casts poured (Figs 5-15 to 5-17). A zirconia framework of an appropriate shade was constructed (Lava, 3M-Espe, Germany) and subsequently veneered with porcelain. The intaglio surface was air abraded with alumina particles and cemented with a self-adhesive resin cement containing an adhesive phosphate monomer (Panavia 21, Kuraray, Japan). The pre- and postoperative results show improved oval-shaped pontics, with correct emergence profiles (Figs 5-18 and 5-21). The lateral incisor abutments have subgingival margins to conceal the dense zirconia–tooth margin interface and harmoniously integrate with the surrounding healthy periodontium. The dento-facial views show the lip line exposing the cervical aspects of the laterals during a relaxed smile. The body shade, cervical chroma, incisal translucency, and characterizations of the FPD blend immaculately with the distal teeth.

5 Traumatic Loss of Maxillary Central Incisors

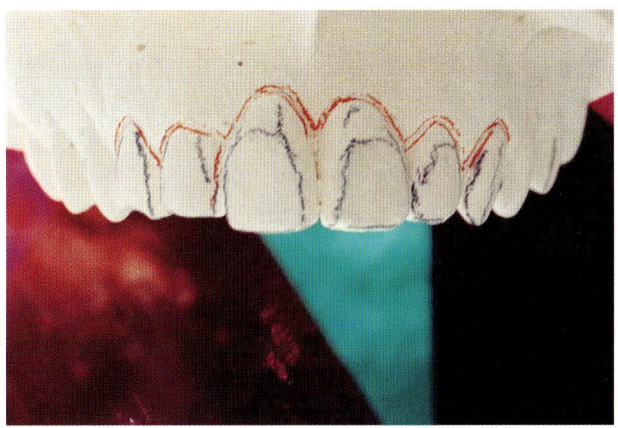

Fig 5-13 Preoperative anterior view of plaster casts with pencil-marked line angles and gingival contours.

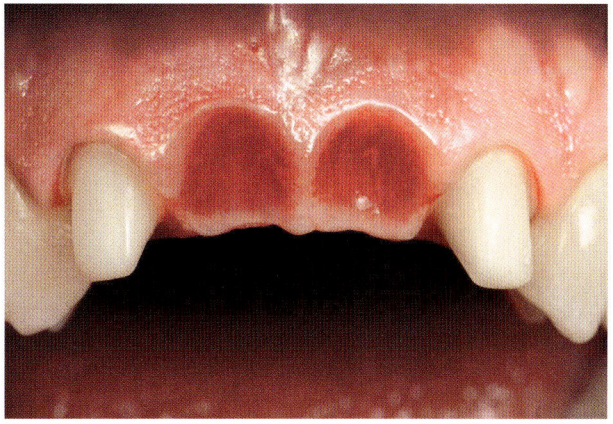

Fig 5-14 Sculpted soft tissue to create ovate shape at central incisor sites.

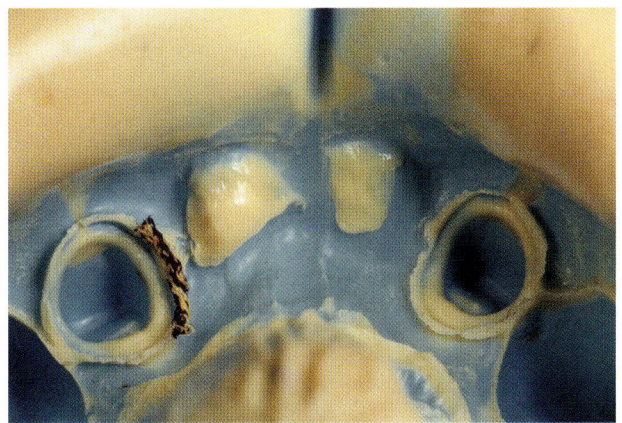

Fig 5-15 Impressions of prepared lateral incisor abutments and sculpted soft tissue at the central incisor sites.

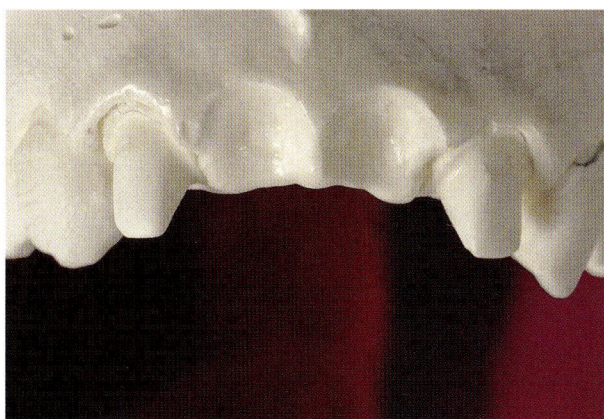

Fig 5-16 Plaster model showing ovate pontic sites: anterior view.

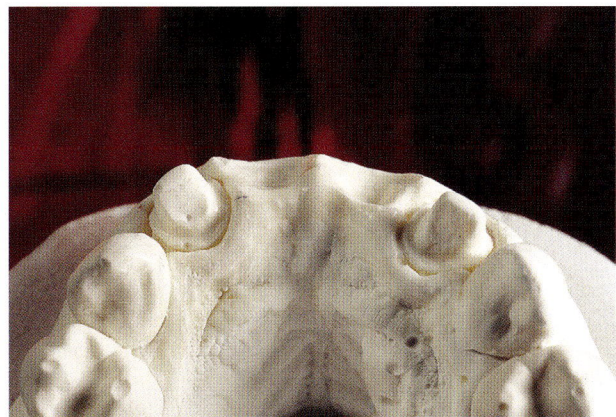

Fig 5-17 Plaster model showing ovate pontic sites: incisal view.

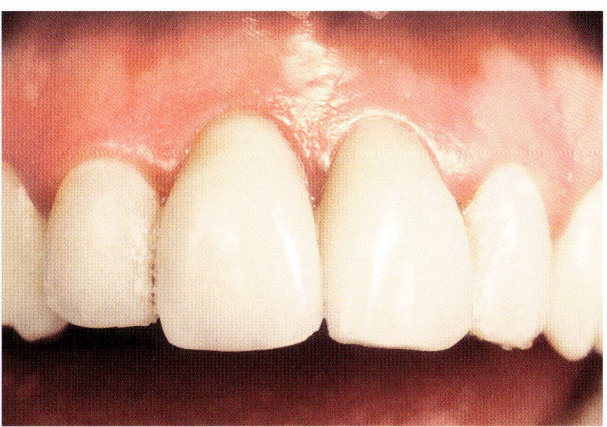

Fig 5-18 Preoperative anterior view.

5 Traumatic Loss of Maxillary Central Incisors

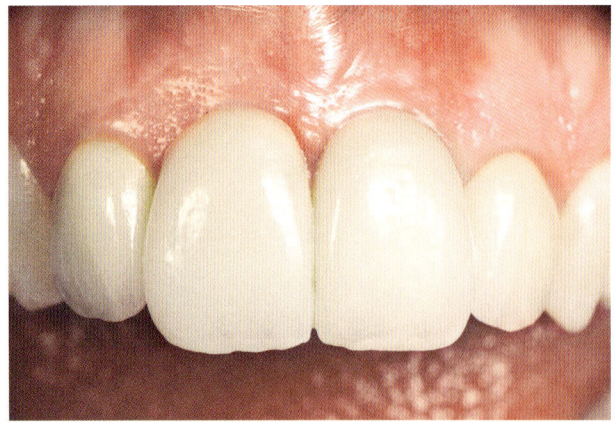

Fig 5-19 Postoperative anterior view.

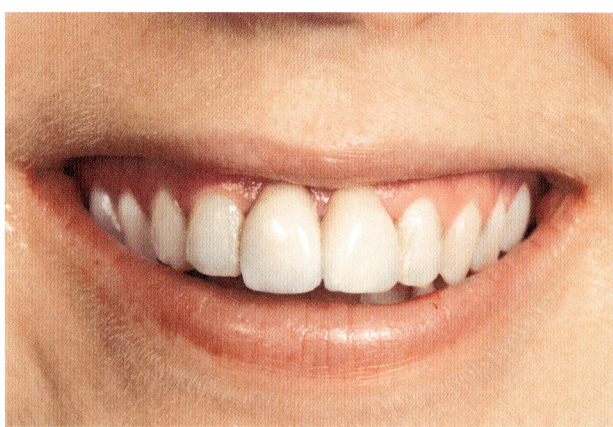

Fig 5-20 Preoperative dento-facial view.

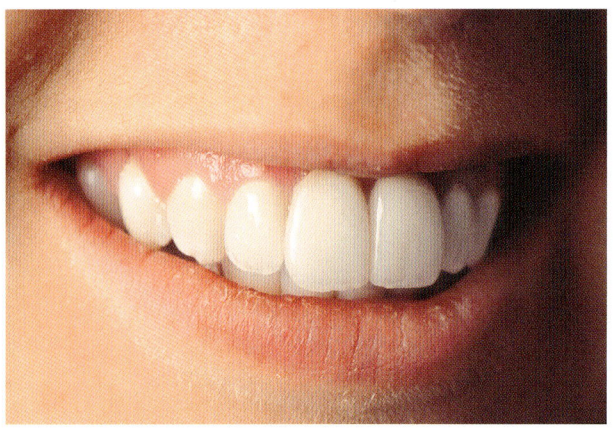

Fig 5-21 Postoperative dento-facial view.

Discussion

The objective of providing a fixed prosthesis with improved esthetics was achieved. The central incisor pontics are perhaps too dominant and could have been slightly narrower and shorter. The disadvantage of this modality was sacrificing two vital teeth as abutments, and the vast horizontal overjet is uncorrected. Owing to the protrusion of the pontics, these are still in a precarious position, and wearing a mouth guard is essential for all contact sports, and especially for swimming!

Vicissitudes of Two Maxillary Incisors Over 21 Years

Laboratory and ceramics: various
Final crowns by Eva Forst, Newbury, UK

Pre- and Postoperative Status

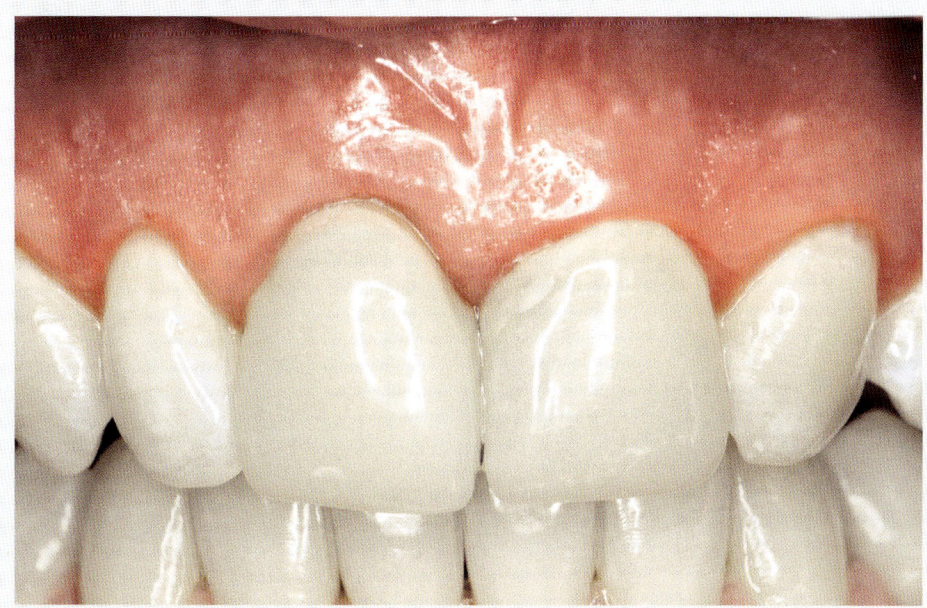

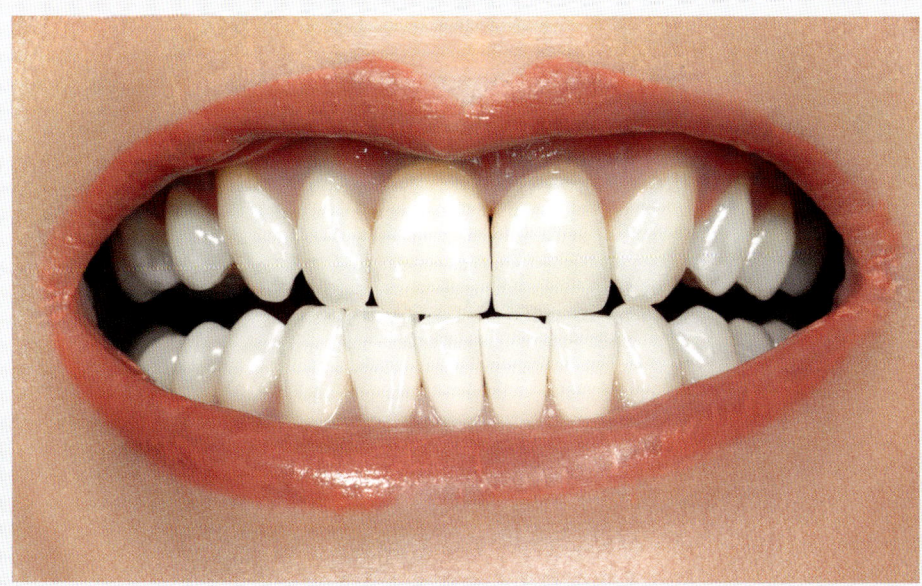

Dental History

The dental history of this young woman spans 21 years, from 1986 to 2007, with the current course of treatment starting in 2006.

In 1986, at the age of 14, the patient was involved in an accident, which resulted in the avulsion and loss of the maxillary left central incisor. To close the residual space, the left lateral incisor was orthodontically moved to occupy the site of the left central incisor. At the same time, the left lateral incisor was provided with a porcelain laminate veneer (PLV) simulating a central incisor tooth.

Several years later, in 1993, the patient attended the practice of the author, complaining of pain from the maxillary right central incisor and expressing concern regarding the appearance of the PLV on the left lateral incisor. A periapical radiograph of the right central incisor, taken on 7 October 1993, revealed that although a defective palatal resin-composite filling was present, presumably sealing an access cavity to the root canal, there was no evidence of an intraradicular filling or apical seal (Fig 6-1). Upon removal of the palatal filling, copious pus exuded from the root canal, which was drained and a course of metronidazole prescribed for 5 days. A few days later, on 14 October, the tooth was symptomless and the root canal sealed with calcium hydroxide and gutta-percha. Unfortunately, the root filling was inadequate, with poor lateral condensation (Fig 6-2). In the meantime, two new PLVs on the right central incisor and the left lateral incisor (simulating the missing left central incisor) were fitted on 12 November 1993. The faulty root filling failed to resolve symptoms from the right central incisor, and on 22 November the gutta-percha was removed and replaced with a palliative dressing. Once symptomless, the canal was sealed with a correctly adapted root filing on 2 December 1993 (Fig 6-3). The open and defective margins of the newly fitted PLVs on the right central and left lateral incisors are clearly discernible on the radiograph.

Two years later, in July 1995, the patient could no longer tolerate the poor esthetics of the PLVs and requested replacements. Additionally, the defective cervical margins of the veneers were encouraging plaque accumulation, their shade was darker than the adjacent teeth, and they had poor shape and characterization, and incorrect texture and luster (Figs 6-4 to 6.8). Notice the left shift of the dental midline compared with the facial midline (Fig 6-5).

Before the veneers were removed, shade analysis was carried out using shade tabs from the Vita Classical shade guide (Figs 6-9 and 6-10). The veneers were sectioned and discarded, the tooth preparations refined (Figs 6-11 and 6-12), and chairside acrylic-resin provisionals were fabricated with improved shape and contours (Figs 6-13 and 6-14). On 22 July 1995, new PLVs were fitted using hydroflouric acid etching and silane to pretreat the intaglio surfaces, and a dentin bonding agent (One-Step, Bisco) with a Vita shade A2 resin-based cement (Ultra-Bond, Ultradent) (Figs 6-15 to 6-17). Although the shape, contour, texture and luster were an improvement, a close inspection (Figs 6-16 and 6-17) revealed that the shade of the PLVs was a

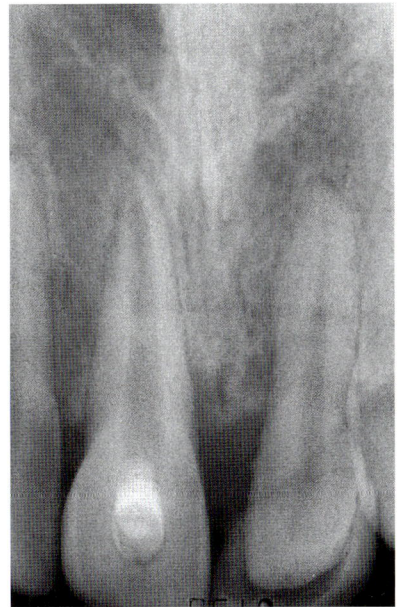

Fig 6-1 7 October 1993: radiograph showing a palatal filling in the maxillary right central incisor without a root filling and a PLV on the adjacent tooth.

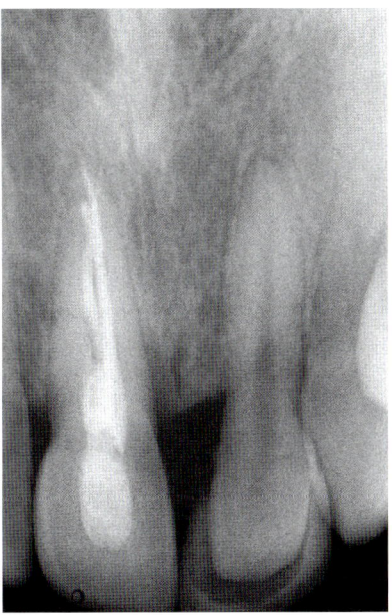

Fig 6-2 14 October 1993: inadequate root filling in the maxillary right central incisor.

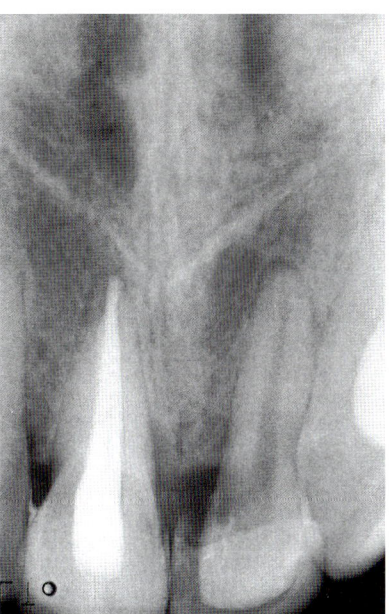

Fig 6-3 2 December 1993: correctly adapted root filling in the maxillary right central incisor, but defective margins of the PLVs are evident.

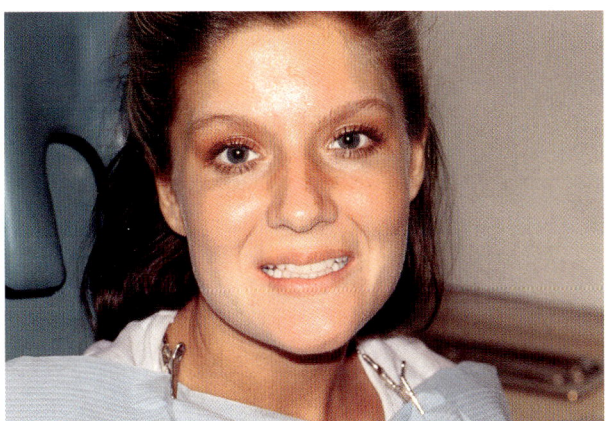

Fig 6-4 July 1995: facial view.

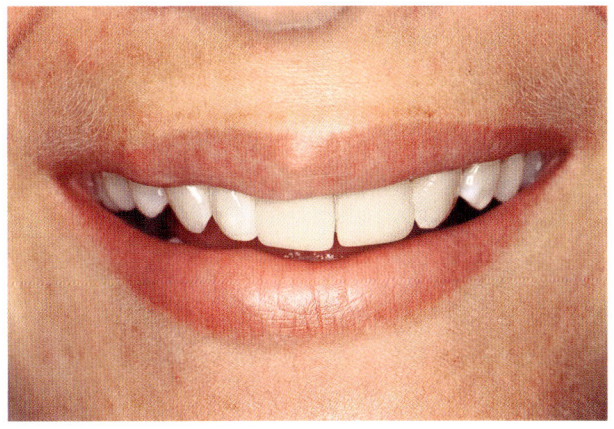

Fig 6-5 July 1995: dento-facial view. Notice the left shift of the dental midline compared with the facial midline.

close match to the mandibular teeth but darker than the adjacent maxillary teeth. Even at a social distance (Fig 6-15), the shade was not perfect.

For the following 2 years, no symptoms were reported, but on 8 May 1997, the patient experienced tenderness at the base of the nose, above the right central incisor. A radiograph revealed a radiolucent apical lesion associated with the right central incisor, which amoxicillin failed to resolve (Fig 6-18). A few days later, the patient was referred to an oral surgeon, with a view to carrying out an apicectomy. This was carried out on 18 June 1997, with concurrent

6 Vicissitudes of Two Maxillary Incisors Over 21 Years

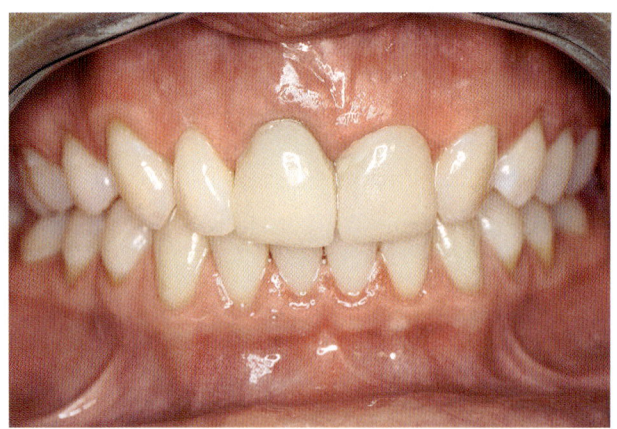

Fig 6-6 July 1995: anterior view showing poor esthetics of the defective PLVs.

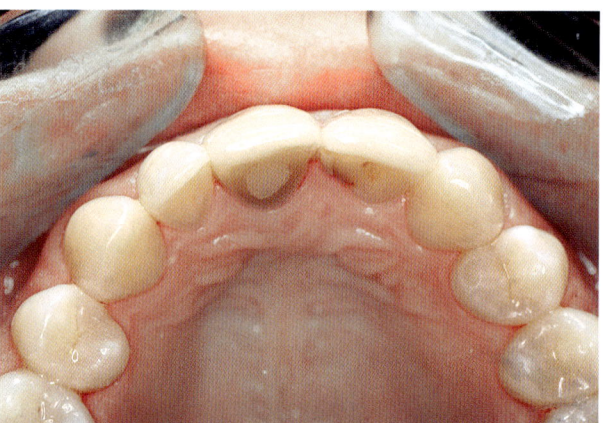

Fig 6-7 July 1995: incisal view.

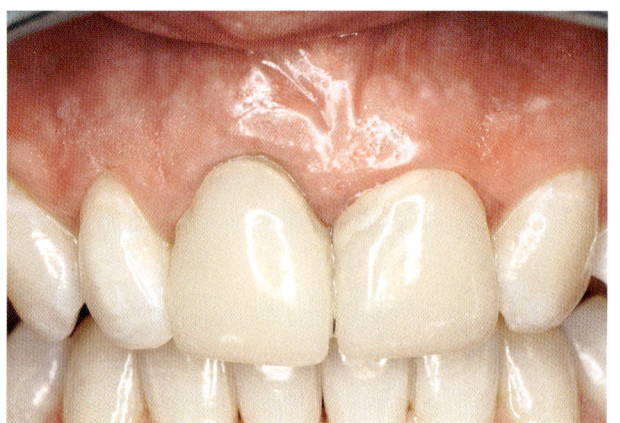

Fig 6-8 July 1995: anterior detailed view, showing the defective margins and poor esthetics of the PLVs.

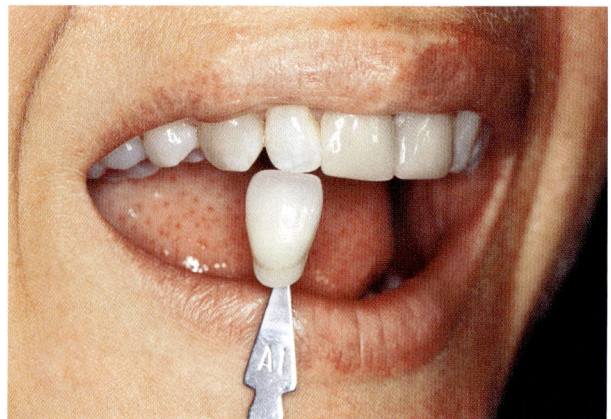

Fig 6-9 July 1995: shade analysis with Vita Classical A1 shade tab.

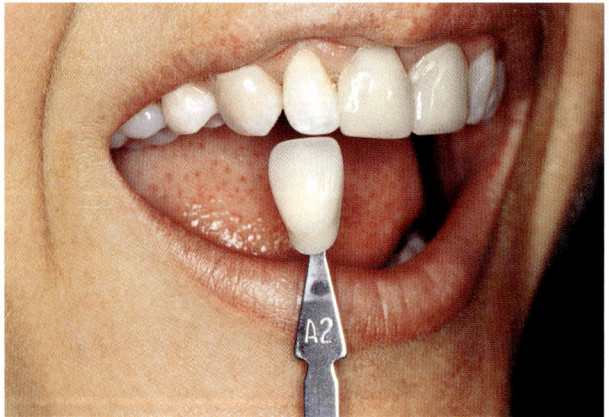

Fig 6-10 July 1995: shade analysis with Vita Classical A2 shade tab.

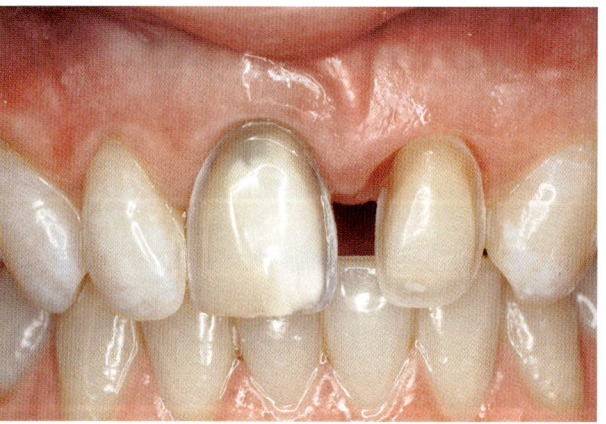

Fig 6-11 July 1995: refined tooth preparations of right central and left lateral incisors.

6 Vicissitudes of Two Maxillary Incisors Over 21 Years

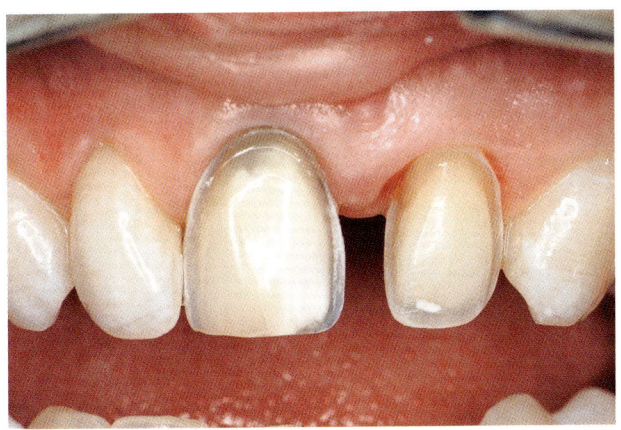

Fig 6-12 July 1995: refined tooth preparations of right central and left lateral incisors.

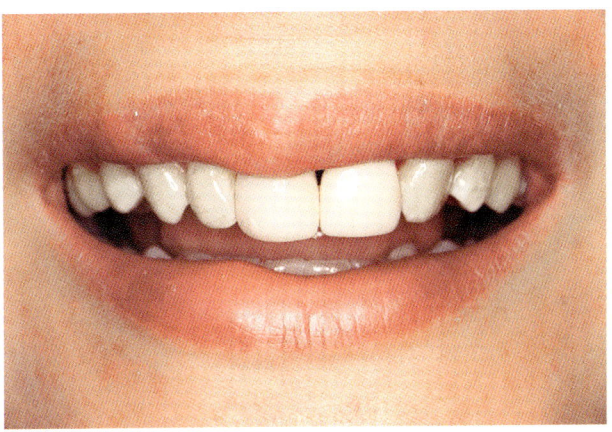

Fig 6-13 July 1995: chairside acrylic-resin provisional veneers on right central and left lateral incisors.

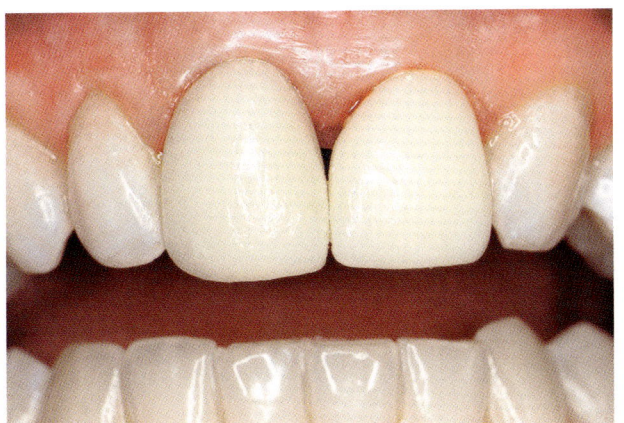

Fig 6-14 July 1995: chairside acrylic-resin provisional veneers on right central and left lateral incisors.

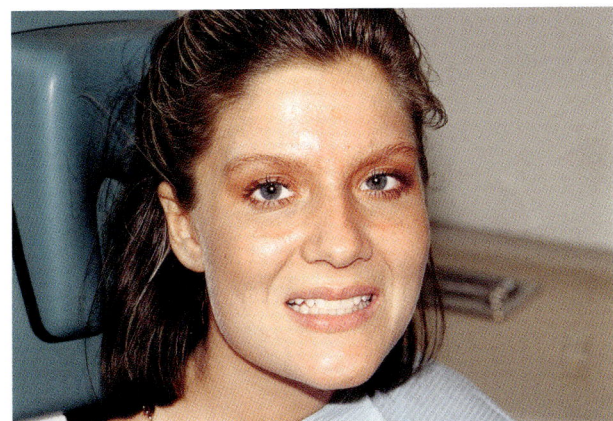

Fig 6-15 July 1995: facial view showing newly cemented PLVs.

retrograde filling as an apical seal (Fig 6-19). The histology report of the curetted apical tissues stated presence of an apical granuloma containing a heavy chronic inflammatory infiltrate. The operation was performed under general anesthesia, which could be questioned as unnecessary for this type of minor surgery, but the patient requested it as she could not bear to endure the procedure with local anesthesia.

Following the apicectomy, the tooth was symptomless for another 2 years. However, on 8 September 1999, the tenderness returned, but this time the radiograph was inconclusive and no substantial apical changes could be detected (Fig 6-20). In addition, an intraoral examination showed absence of a sinus or erythema. The cause of the recurring symptoms was most likely residual bacteria at the apex of the root. A course of amoxicillin was successful at relieving all symptoms, and abated the infection for the next 6 years.

6 Vicissitudes of Two Maxillary Incisors Over 21 Years

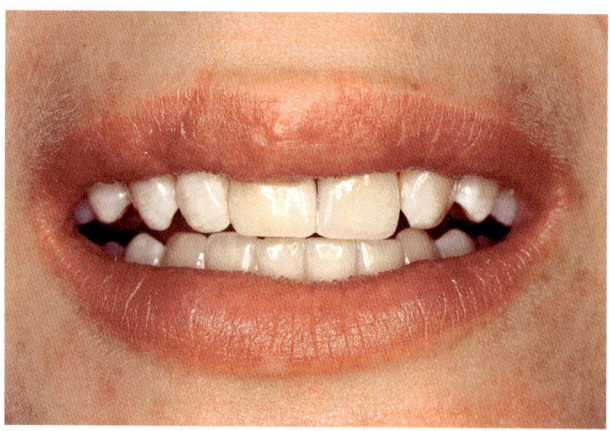

Fig 6-16 July 1995: dento-facial view showing newly cemented PLVs. Notice that the veneers are darker than the adjacent natural maxillary dentition.

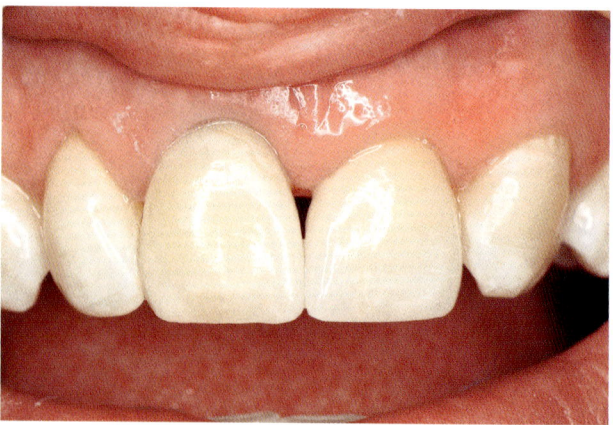

Fig 6-17 July 1995: anterior view showing newly cemented PLVs.

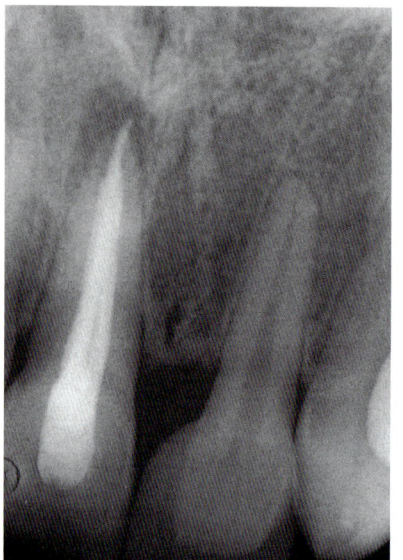

Fig 6-18 May 1997: apical radiolucent area associated with the right central incisor.

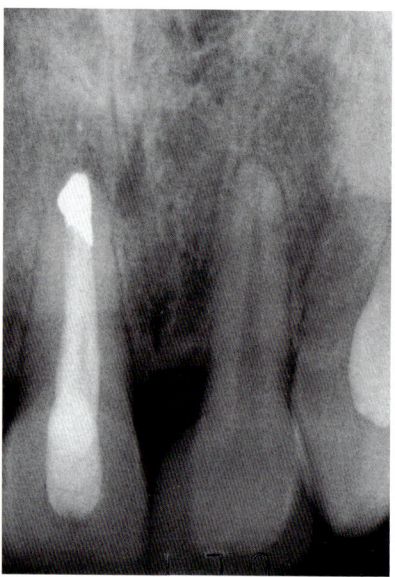

Fig 6-19 June 1997: retrograde apical seal following apicectomy of the right central incisor.

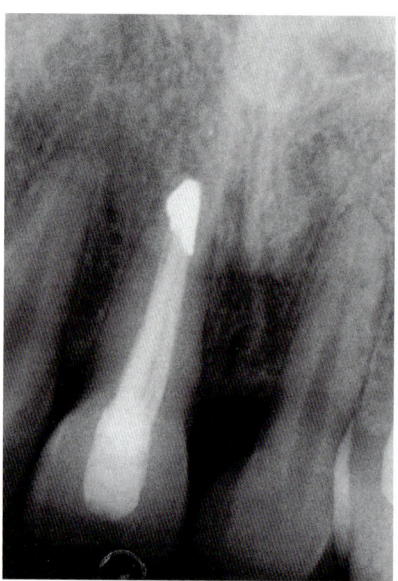

Fig 6-20 September 1999: no apparent changes in apical region of the right central incisor compared with June 1997.

In the interim period, the right central incisor was progressively discoloring, and the darkened root was becoming increasingly visible through the thin periodontium (Figs 6-21 and 6-22). Besides the discoloration, which was only apparent during an exaggerated smile (Fig 6-23), the patient was concerned that the veneer on the left "central" incisor was slightly longer than the right central incisor (Fig 6-24). To satisfy her wishes, a series of photographs was taken in June 2004 to appraise her anterior dental esthetics (Figs 6-25 to 6-31). Recall that when the veneers were fitted in 1995 (Figs 6-15 to 6-17), their shade was darker than the adjacent maxillary teeth. But 9 years on, the

6 Vicissitudes of Two Maxillary Incisors Over 21 Years

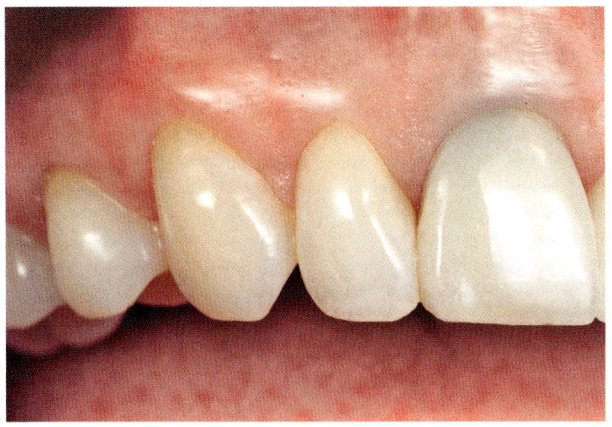

Fig 6-21 June 2004: right lateral view showing visibility of the discolored root of the right central incisor through the thin periodontium.

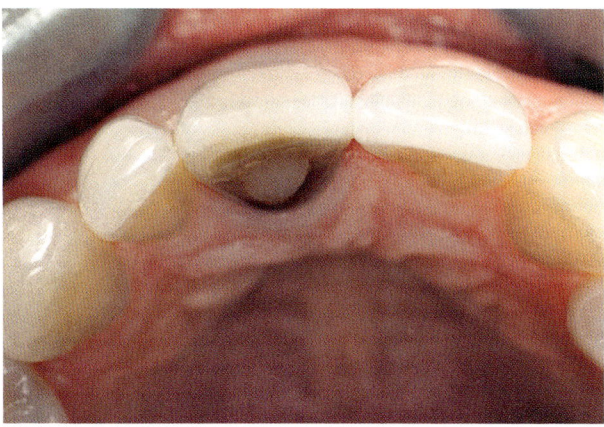

Fig 6-22 June 2004: incisal view showing the heavily discolored right central incisor.

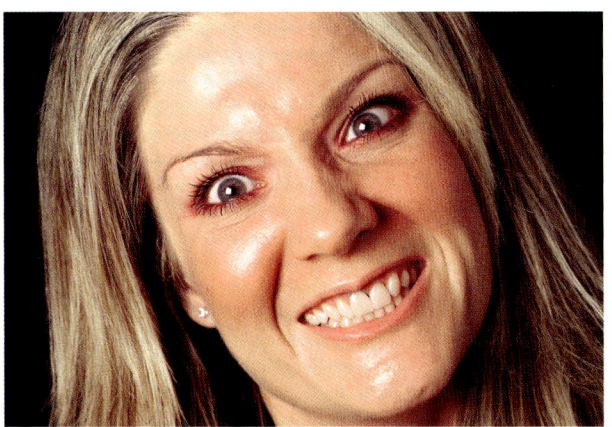

Fig 6-23 June 2004: visibility of the discolored cervical margin of the right central incisor during an exaggerated smile.

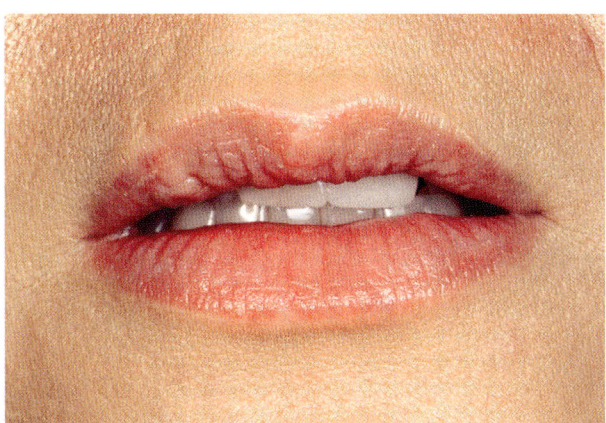

Fig 6-24 June 2004: dento-facial view with lips at habitual "rest" position showing that the left "central" veneer is longer than the right counterpart.

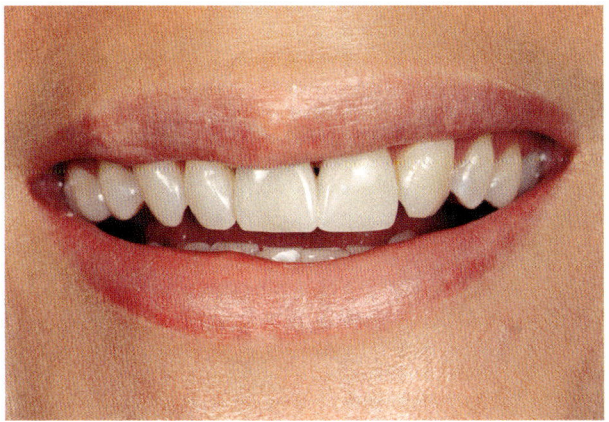

Fig 6-25 June 2004: dento-facial view during a relaxed smile.

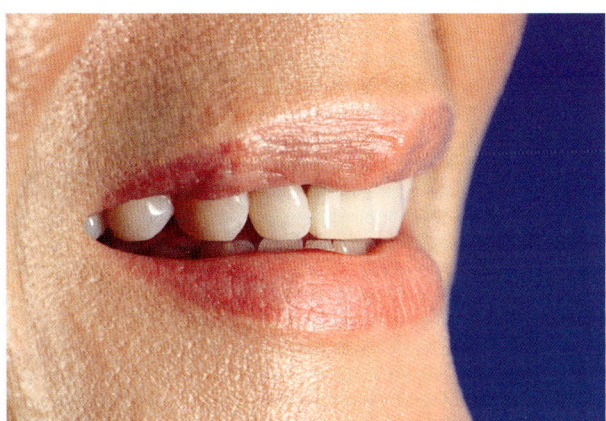

Fig 6-26 June 2004: right lateral dento-facial view during a relaxed smile.

6 Vicissitudes of Two Maxillary Incisors Over 21 Years

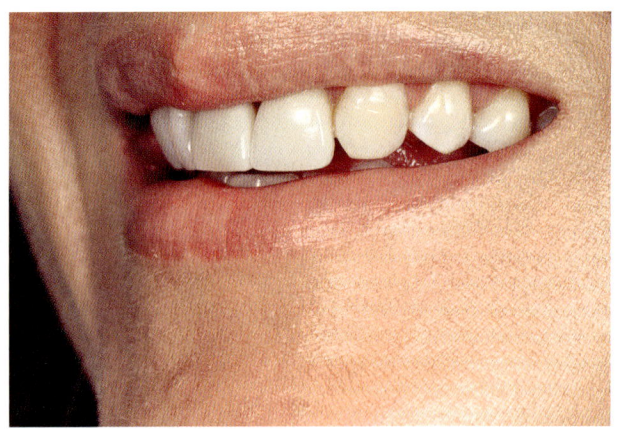

Fig 6-27 June 2004: left lateral dento-facial view during a relaxed smile. Notice that the PLV on the left "central" incisor appears to be hanging down.

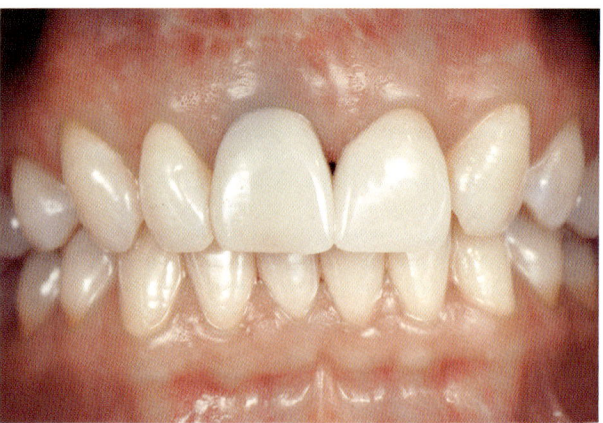

Fig 6-28 June 2004: anterior view in centric occlusion.

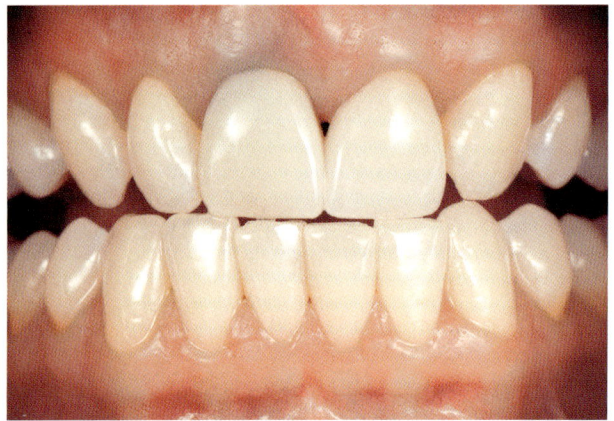

Fig 6-29 June 2004: anterior view in protrusion.

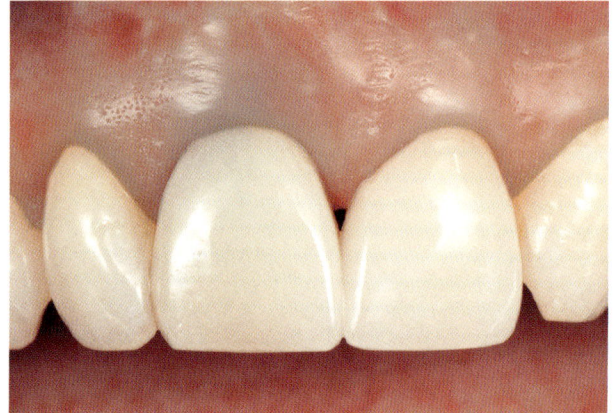

Fig 6-30 June 2004: anterior view showing cervical discoloration around the PLV on the right central incisor.

natural teeth had chromatically aged, and loss of surface staining on the Empress laminates had allowed the veneers to blend with the adjacent dentition. Also, the median interproximal papilla was more coronal than in 1995 (compare Figs 6-17 and 6-30), but it could never completely fill the interdental space since the interproximal bone crest was flat (visible in the preceding radiographs), and the distance from its most apical aspect to the contact point was greater than 5 mm.

It is debatable whether the left veneer was longer, and the discrepancy was unnoticeable during smiling. The illusion of increased length was caused by the tooth distal to the left veneer being a canine, not a lateral incisor. Hence,

6 Vicissitudes of Two Maxillary Incisors Over 21 Years

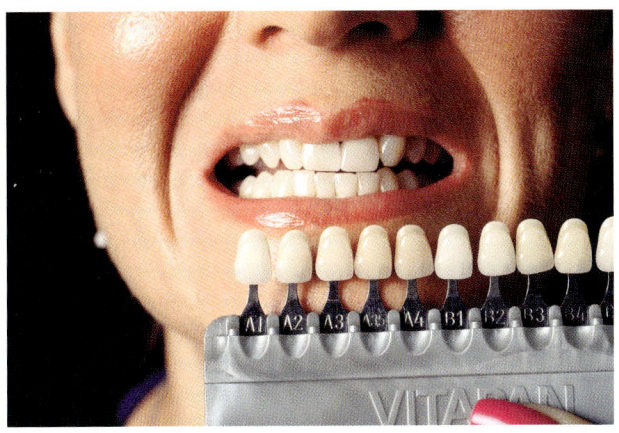

Fig 6-31 June 2004: shade analysis using the Vita Classical shade guide.

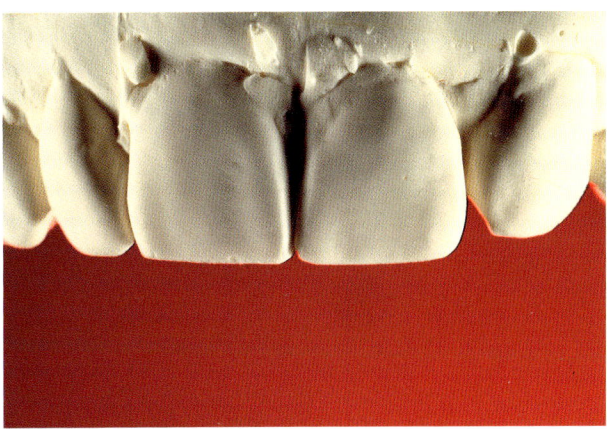

Fig 6-32 June 2004: plaster cast of existing PLVs.

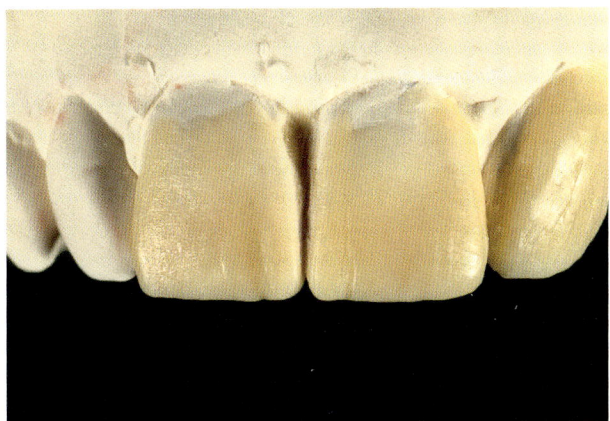

Fig 6-33 June 2004: diagnostic waxup of proposed restorations on the left "central" incisor and left canine (simulating a left lateral incisor).

the incisal embrasure was exaggerated, giving the appearance of a longer veneer. To satisfy the patient's concerns, a diagnostic waxup was carried out on 5 June 2004, simulating the left canine as a lateral to correct this apparent anomaly (Figs 6-32 and 6-33). After discussing the "pros and cons" of filing down the canine for another veneer or crown, the patient was dissuaded from pursuing this destructive option, which would have resulted in negligible esthetic gain.

In December 2005, the lingering infection associated with the right central incisor returned once more. This was the starting point of the current course of treatment.

Preoperative Status

On 21 December 2005, the patient attended with a buccal swelling above the right central incisor. A periapical radiograph showed a small radiolucency at its apex (Fig 6-34), and a 7-day course of metronidazole alleviated the swelling during the Christmas festivities. In the new year, the patient consulted the oral surgeon who had performed the original apicectomy in 1997. He suggested that since the tooth had survived for nearly 9 years after the first apicectomy, a similar procedure might have comparable success. However, the patient was weary at the thought of another apicectomy, possibly with general anesthesia, and she requested a second opinion. An appointment was sought with an implantologist, who suggested that an apicectomy could result in gingival recession as a consequence of raising a muco-periosteal flap, which given the presence of root discoloration might further compromise esthetics. His advice was to extract the right central incisor, provide a transitional acrylic-resin removable denture, and, following a period of healing, consider an implant.

Treatment Options

1. Second apicectomy of the right central incisor with extensive curettage to clear residual and resilient bacteria (Fig 6-35).
2. Extract the right central incisor and replace with an acrylic-resin removable partial denture (Fig 6-36).
3. Extract the right central incisor and restore the space with cantilever bridge using the left lateral as an abutment (with or without a palatal wing on the right lateral) (Fig 6-37).
4. Three-unit fixed partial denture, using the right and left lateral incisors as abutments (Fig 6-38).
5. Extract the right central incisor and replace with an implant-supported crown (Fig 6-39).

Scientific Credence for Treatment Options

The "pros and cons" of another apicectomy have been outlined above. The partial denture would be predicable, but it would be prone to dislodgment, and future recession at the pontic site would require periodic relining or replacement. The cantilever bridge would be unstable, prone to rotation and dislodgement (certainly without a palatal wing on a contralateral tooth), but it would be less invasive than the fixed partial denture option, which is highly destructive. The implant option would obviously resolve the discolored root "shine through", but a thin biotype makes surgery precarious, often predisposing to postoperative gingival recession. Furthermore, the meager blood supply to the site after recurrent infections would necessitate two or more surgical stages, strategically timed to allow new blood vessels to colonize the area.

6 Vicissitudes of Two Maxillary Incisors Over 21 Years

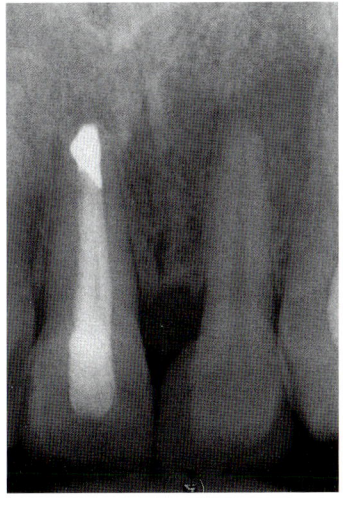

Fig 6-34 December 2005: radiograph showing the apical lesion associated with the right central incisor.

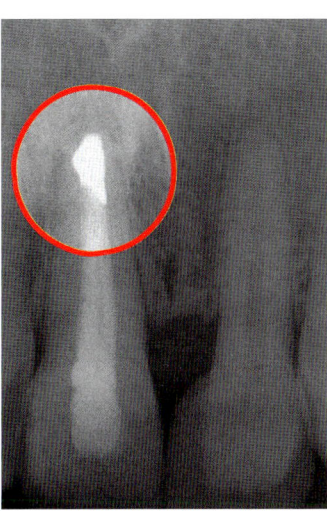

Fig 6-35 Option 1: second apicectomy of the right central incisor with extensive curettage.

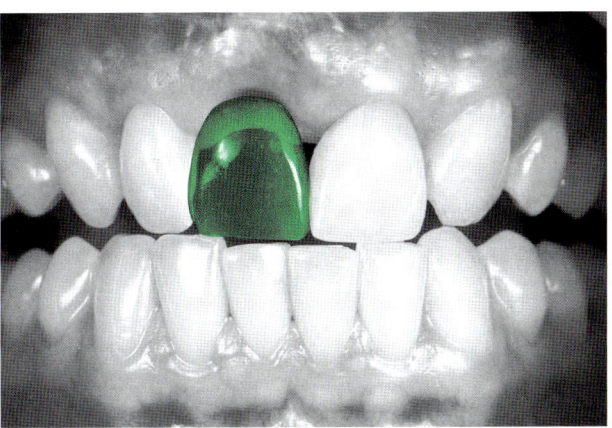

Fig 6-36 Option 2: acrylic-resin removable partial denture (green).

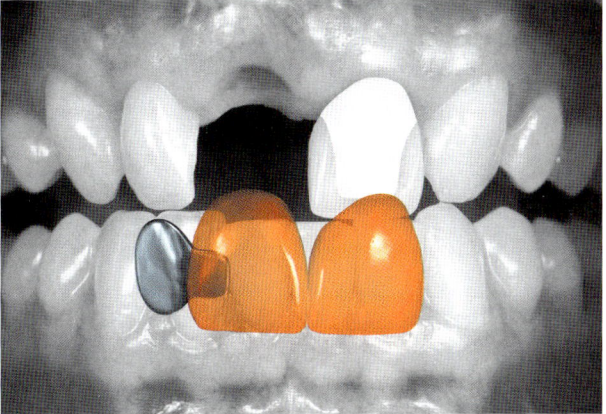

Fig 6-37 Option 3: cantilever bridge (orange) with palatal wing, using the left lateral as an abutment.

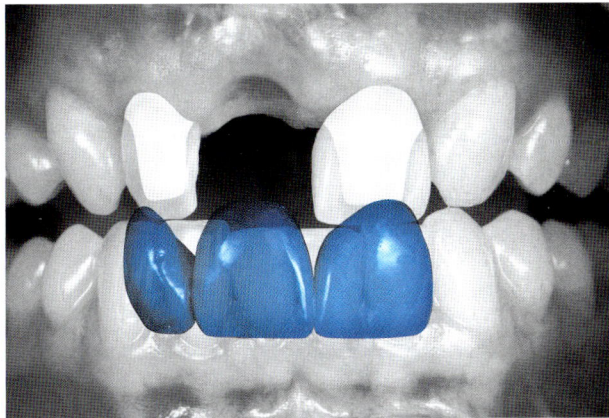

Fig 6-38 Option 4: three-unit fixed partial denture (blue), using the right lateral and left central incisors as abutments.

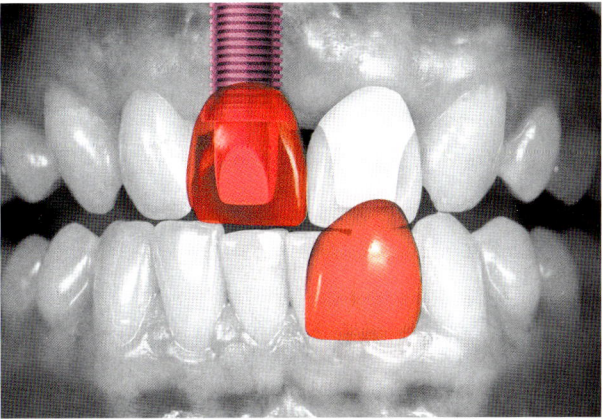

Fig 6-39 Option 5: implant-supported crown (red), and a new crown on the left central incisor.

73

Clinical Erudition and Feasibility

The apicectomy would require an experienced surgeon for delicate tissue manipulation to minimize trauma to the thin biotype. The denture and bridge options were straightforward, and within the remit of the practitioner. The implant option would require experience to extract the central incisor atraumatically without damaging the thin and fragile buccal bone plate. Furthermore, if recession ensued, connective tissue grafting from the palate would be a necessity.

Patient Needs and Wants

Although the patient was ambivalent about the apicectomy versus implant options, after careful deliberation she refused the former. She was also loathed to wear a removable denture and rejected the fixed partial denture and cantilever bridge options as too destructive and with potential future risks of endodontic complications. She opted for the implant option, with the understanding that treatment would be protracted and costly, and that the esthetics would be limited by postsurgical gingival recession, which would probably be insignificant owing to her low lip line (see Fig 6-25).

In addition, the patient wished to bleach her teeth to overcome the chromatic aging prior to any new restorations. To match the postbleaching shade, the PLV on the left lateral incisor (simulating the central incisor) would also require replacement (possibly with a crown). Finally, she also requested periodontal plastic surgery to achieve symmetry of the gingival zeniths around the two new restorations. As previously stated, achieving equal gingival zeniths is not necessary, but the patient requested this procedure as part of the treatment plan.

Treatment Sequence

The first stage was to extract the right central incisor, which was carried out on 17 March 2006 using periotomes and taking care not to damage the buccal bone plate. Concurrently, using the bio-col technique, the socket was grafted with Bio-Oss and sealed with Bio-Oss Collagen. A transitional acrylic-resin removable partial denture was immediately inserted to prevent dislodgement of the grafting materials. The acrylic-resin tooth on the denture was trimmed to support and sculpt the soft tissues. Photographs taken on 29 April 2006 show the healing socket, sculptured tissue, and the denture in situ (Figs 6-40 to 6-45). Three months later, on 28 July 2006, maintenance of soft and hard tissue architecture was apparent (Figs 6-46 and 6-47), and a radiograph showed integration of the grafting materials (Fig 6-48).

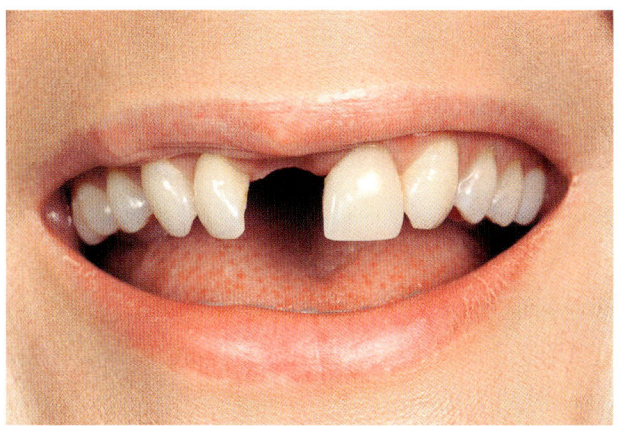

Fig 6-40 April 2006: dento-facial view following extraction of the right central incisor.

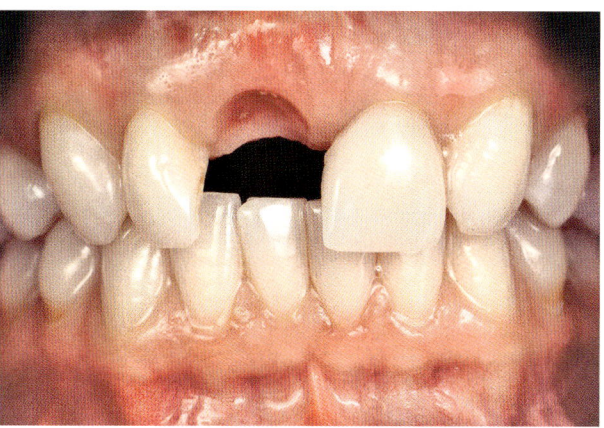

Fig 6-41 April 2006: anterior view in centric occlusion.

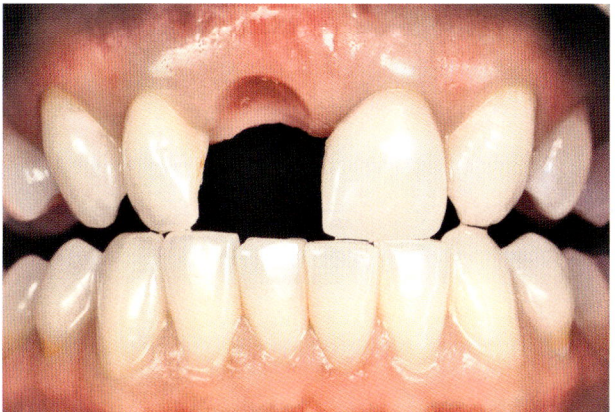

Fig 6-42 April 2006: anterior view in protrusion.

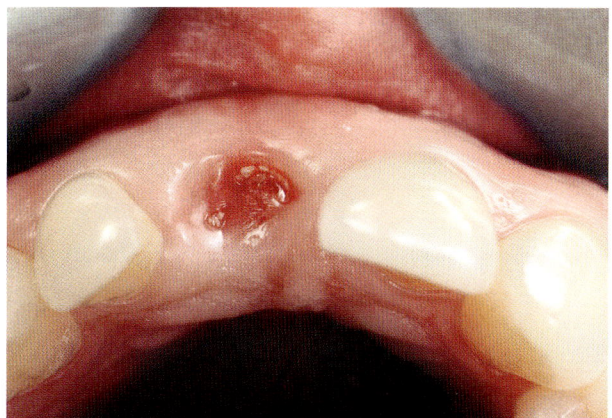

Fig 6-43 April 2006: incisal view of the grafted site. Notice the remnants of grafting material in the healing socket.

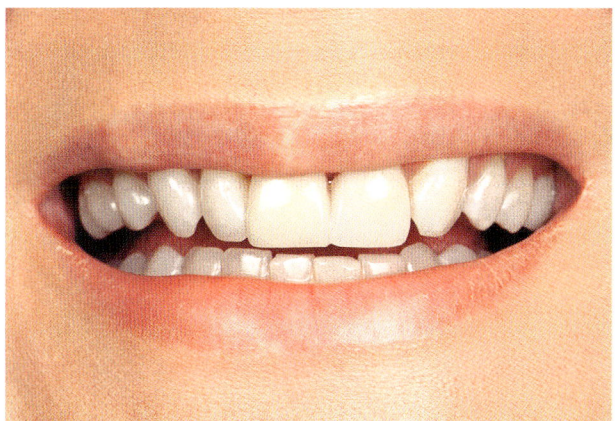

Fig 6-44 April 2006: dento-facial view with the acrylic-resin provisional denture in situ to replace the missing right central incisor.

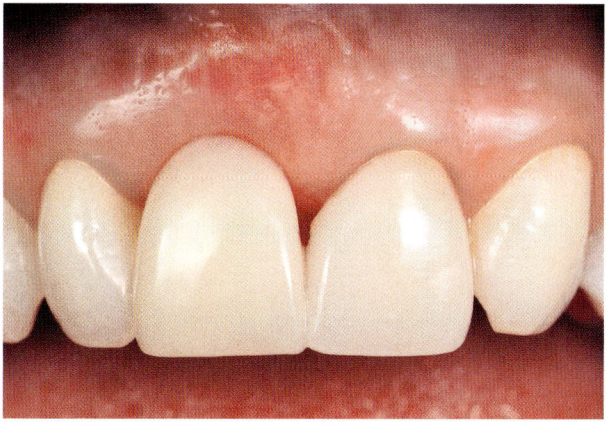

Fig 6-45 April 2006: anterior view with the acrylic-resin provisional denture in situ to sculpt the extraction site at the right central incisor region.

6 Vicissitudes of Two Maxillary Incisors Over 21 Years

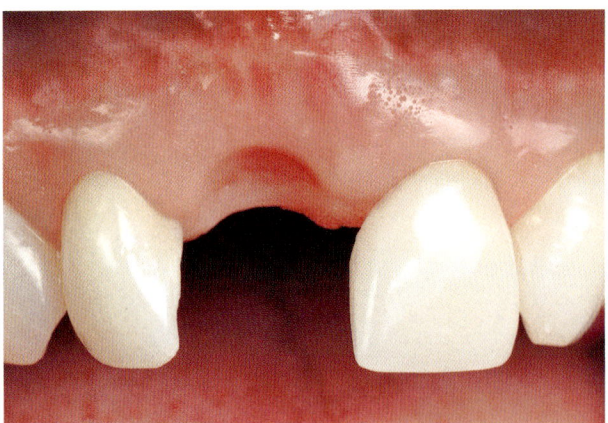

Fig 6-46 July 2006: anterior view showing tissue maturation at the extraction site.

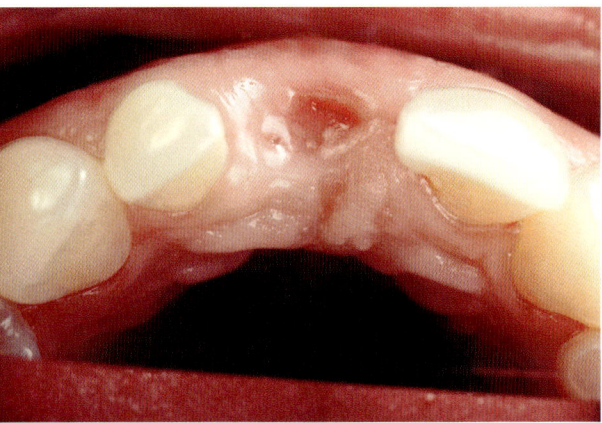

Fig 6-47 July 2006: incisal view showing tissue maturation at the extraction site. Notice that grafting immediately after extraction has prevented collapse of the buccal tissue architecture.

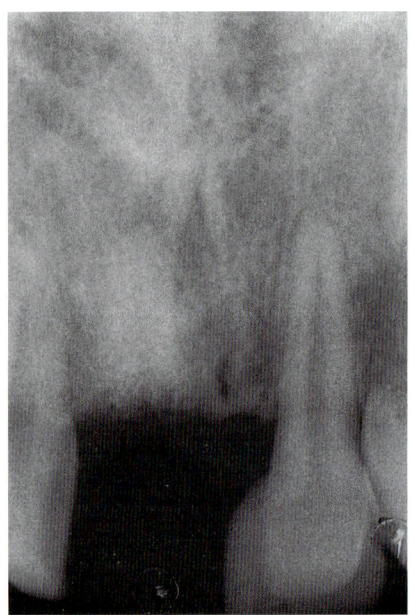

Fig 6-48 July 2006: radiograph showing integration of the grafting material at the right central incisor site.

The site was allowed to mature for a further 10 weeks. During that time, an impression was made for a diagnostic waxup of the right central incisor (Figs 6-49 and 6-50). From the waxup, a stent was fabricated to guide fixture placement (Figs 6-51 and 6-52). An appointment was scheduled for fixture placement on 19 October 2006 (after the summer holidays). The 7-month healing period, from March to October, was essential to allow vascularization of the potential implant site.

The surgery protocol was as follows. First, it was decided to carry out a flapless procedure to minimize the possibility of postsurgical recession owing to the thin biotype. Second, immediate temporarization of the implant was opted

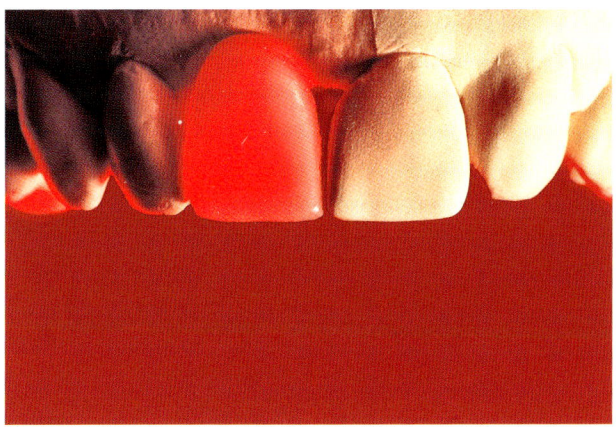

Fig 6-49 July 2006: anterior view of the diagnostic waxup of the right central incisor.

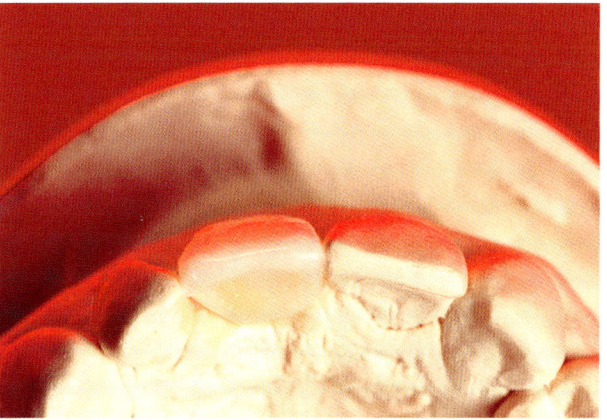

Fig 6-50 July 2006: incisal view of the diagnostic waxup of the right central incisor.

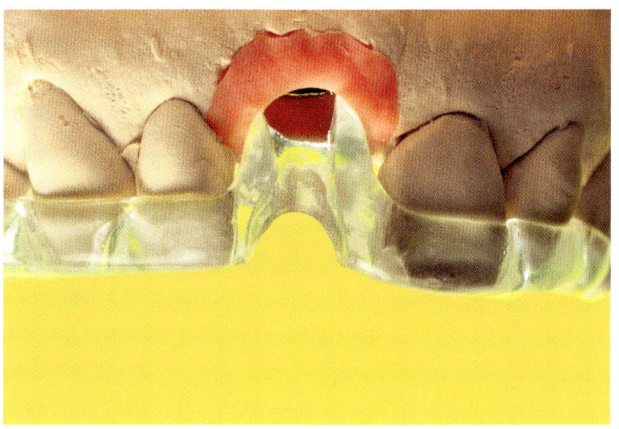

Fig 6-51 July 2006: anterior view of the surgical stent for the right central incisor implant.

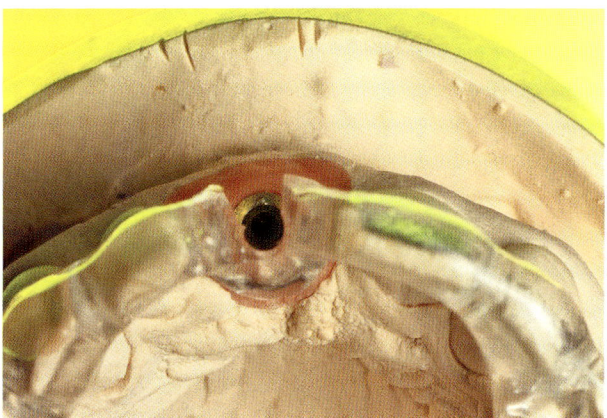

Fig 6-52 July 2006: incisal view of the surgical stent for the right central incisor implant.

for because the patient disliked the removable denture, and because a fixed temporary crown would be more stable for sculpting the transmucosal tissue around the implant.

Using the surgical stent as a guide for osteotomy and positioning of the implant, a RP 4.3 mm NobelReplace fixture (Nobel Biocare, Sweden) was placed. Primary stability was achieved and a healing cap screwed on to the fixture head. On the same day, the patient returned for a fixture level impression (Fig 6-53), and the denture was trimmed and relined (Fig 6-54) to fit over the healing cap while awaiting a laboratory-fabricated temporary crown (Figs 6-55 to 6-58). The occlusion of the denture was cleared to avoid undue stresses on the implant fixture.

6 Vicissitudes of Two Maxillary Incisors Over 21 Years

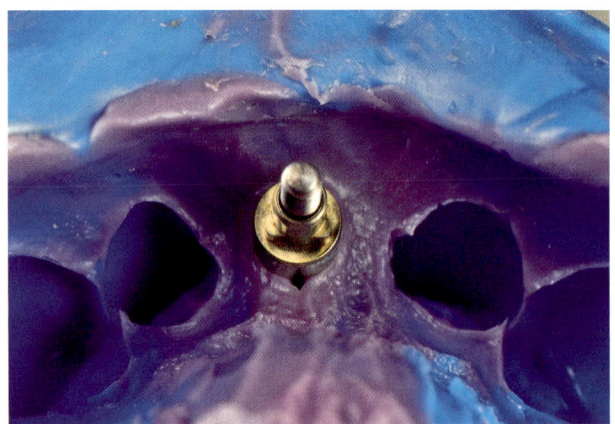

Fig 6-53 19 October 2006: fixture level impression.

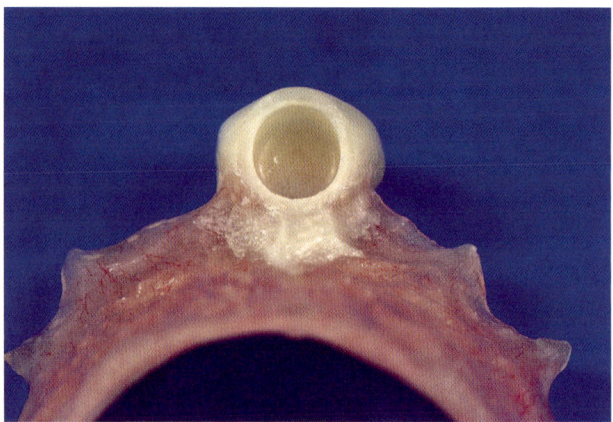

Fig 6-54 19 October 2006: acrylic-resin partial denture modified to fit over the healing cap.

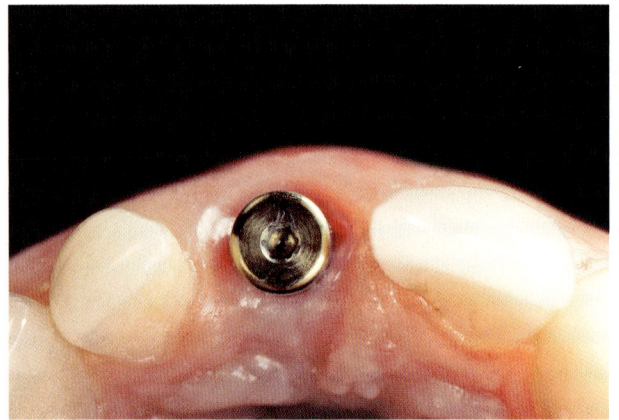

Fig 6-55 19 October 2006: incisal view of the healing cap.

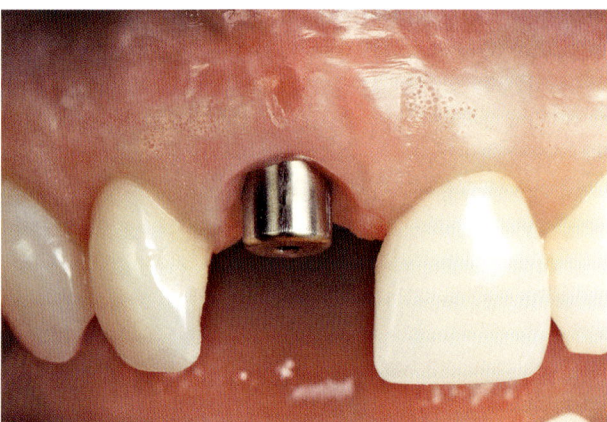

Fig 6-56 19 October 2006: anterior view of the healing cap.

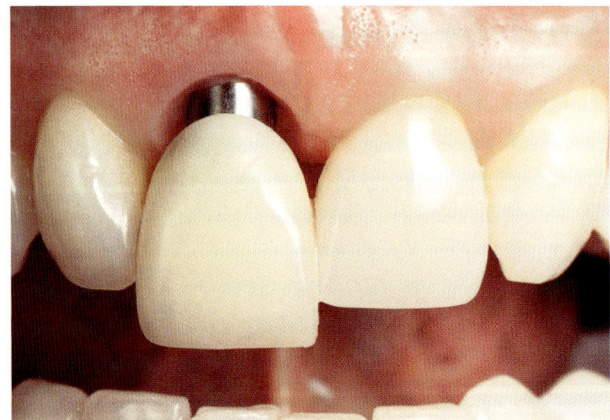

Fig 6-57 19 October 2006: denture being placed onto the healing cap.

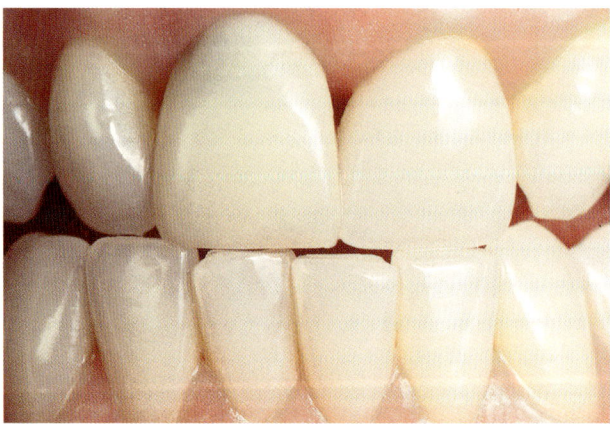

Fig 6-58 19 October 2006: denture fully seated over the healing cap.

6 Vicissitudes of Two Maxillary Incisors Over 21 Years

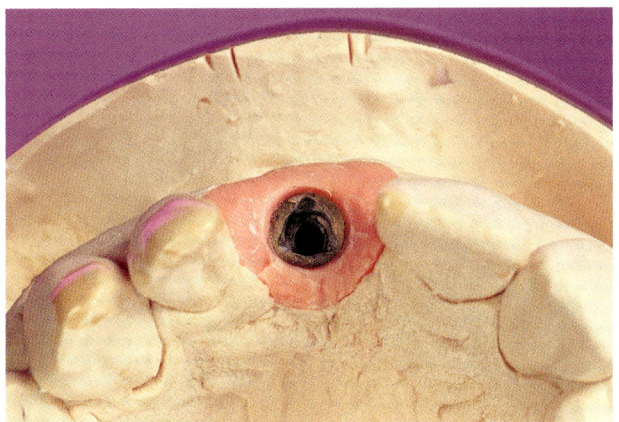

Fig 6-59 October 2006: incisal view of implant analogue with soft tissue model.

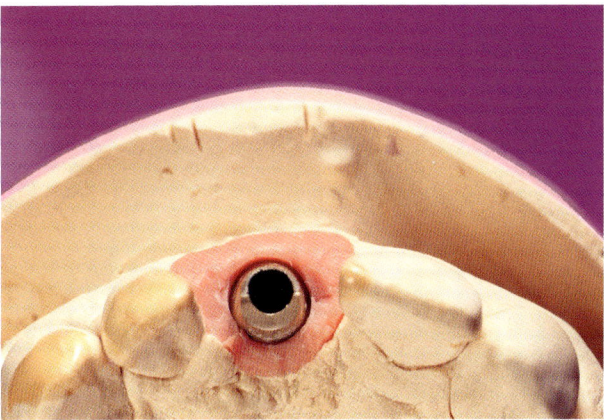

Fig 6-60 October 2006: incisal view of the trimmed titanium abutment for the cement-retained provisional crown.

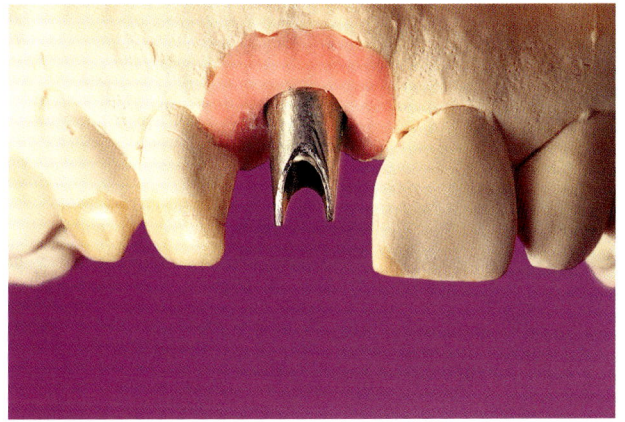

Fig 6-61 October 2006: anterior view of the trimmed titanium abutment for the cement-retained provisional crown.

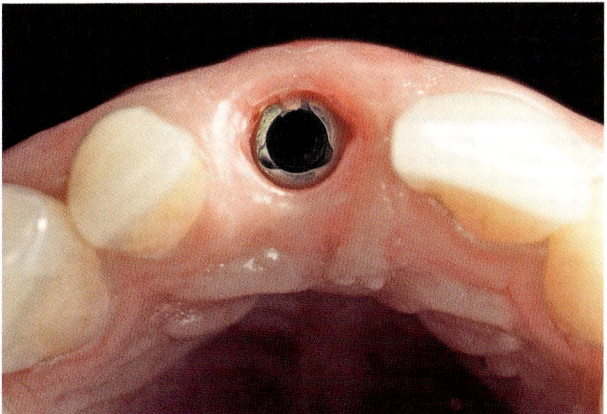

Fig 6-62 25 October 2006: incisal view of the implant fixture.

In the dental laboratory, a plaster model was cast using an implant analogue with silicone soft tissue to simulate the gingival architecture. A titanium abutment was trimmed and polished to support a cement-retained temporary crown (Figs 6-59 to 6-61). On 25 October 2006, the healing cap was removed, the titanium abutment fitted, and the screw access hole blocked with a cotton wool pellet and temporary dressing material. The temporary crown, fabricated of resin composite (HFO Enamel, Optident, UK), was cemented using zinc oxide-eugenol transitional cement (Fig 6-62 and 6-67).

While the implant was integrating (Fig 6-68), the reminder of the treatment was carried out. On 24 January 2007, crown lengthening was performed around the left lateral incisor. Pictures taken a month later, on 28 February 2007, show that the position of the free gingival margin (FGM) around the left lateral incisor was more apical than anticipated (Fig 6-69). In order to replace

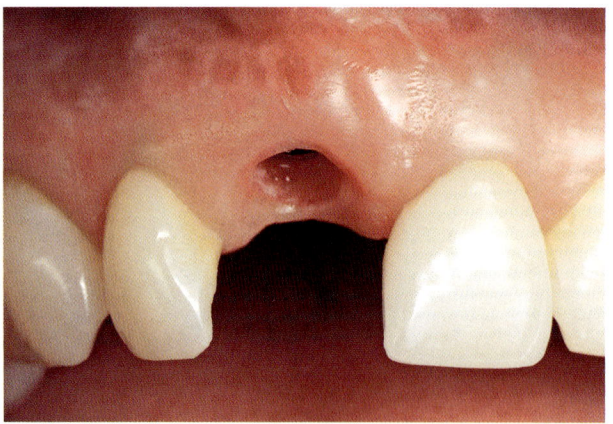

Fig 6-63 25 October 2006: anterior view of the implant fixture.

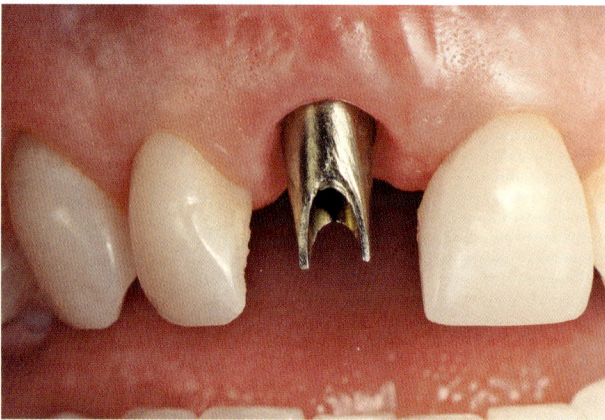

Fig 6-64 25 October 2006: anterior view of the titanium abutment.

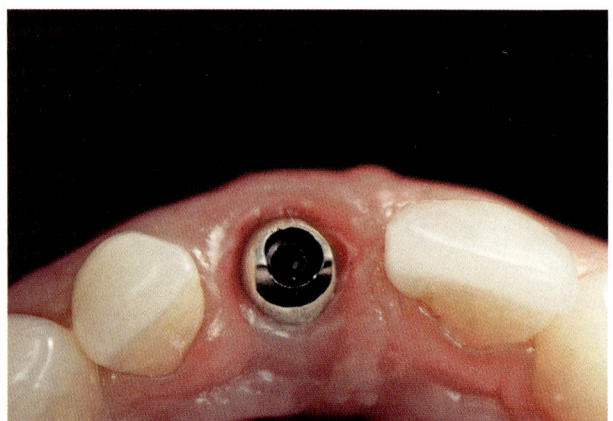

Fig 6-65 25 October 2006: incisal view of the titanium abutment.

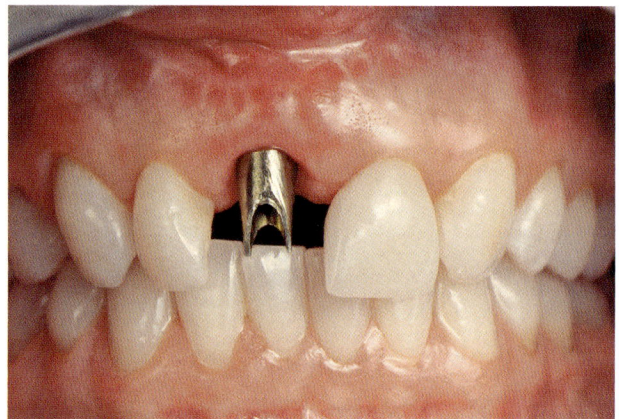

Fig 6-66 25 October 2006: verifying occlusion with the titanium abutment.

the PLV, the left lateral incisor was prepared for a full-coverage crown, and a week later, on 9 March, a laboratory-fabricated resin-composite temporary crown was fitted. The decision to provide a crown instead of another PLV was empirical. Furthermore, because of the low lip line, crown lengthening could be regarded as superfluous. But the patient requested this procedure, claiming that during an exaggerated smile the gingival zeniths of the centrals were visible (Figs 6-70 and 6-71).

Two months after crown lengthening, on 23 March 2007, the discrepancy between the right and left gingival zeniths was 1 mm, allowing visibility of the left lateral root apical to the finish line (Figs 6-72 to 6-75). The gingivae were allowed to heal further, with the possibility of coronal rebound of the FGM. However, after a further 2 months the situation was unchanged. At this juncture, the patient was offered the choice of either accepting the position of the FGM and moving the crown margin subgingivally, or attempting another surgical

6 Vicissitudes of Two Maxillary Incisors Over 21 Years

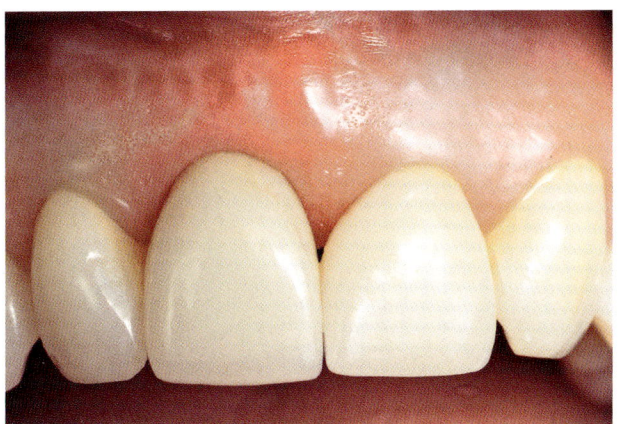

Fig 6-67 25 October 2006: provisional crown cemented over the titanium abutment at the right central incisor site.

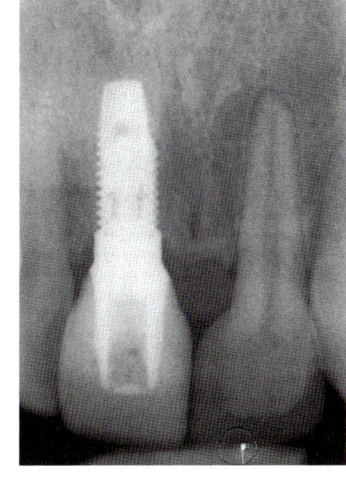

Fig 6-68 January 2007: radiograph showing successful integration of the implant.

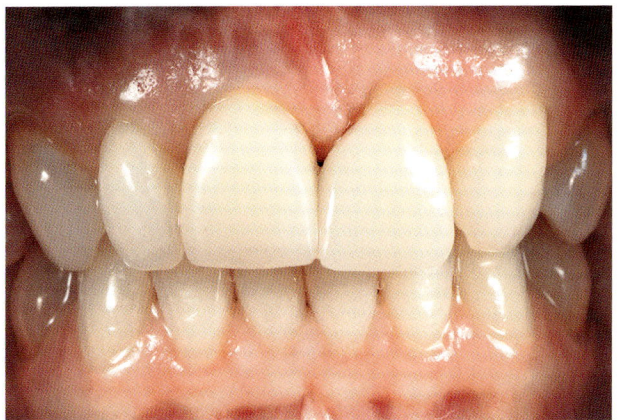

Fig 6-69 February 2007: the FGM after crown lengthening around the left lateral incisor is more apical compared with the right central incisor site.

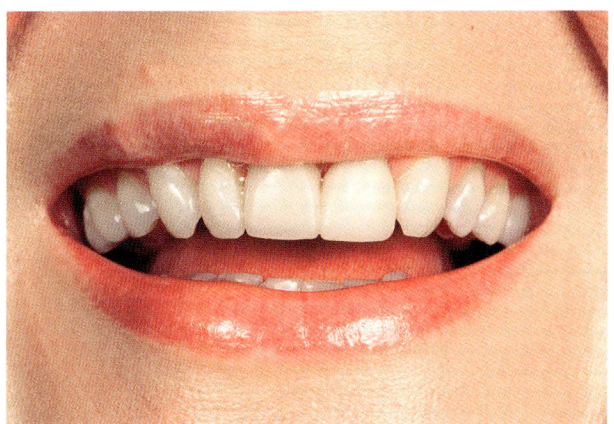

Fig 6-70 9 March 2007: dento-facial view during a relaxed smile.

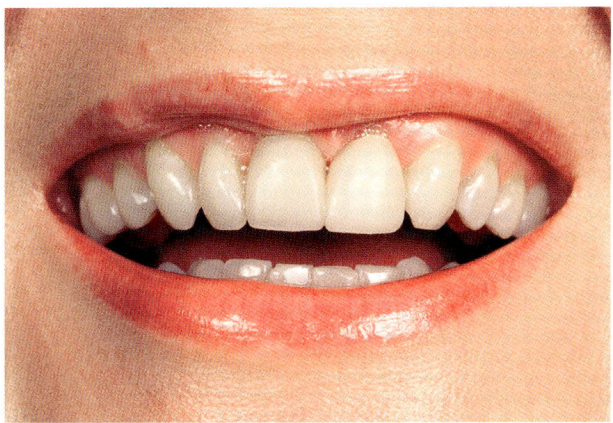

Fig 6-71 9 March 2007: dento-facial view during an exaggerated smile.

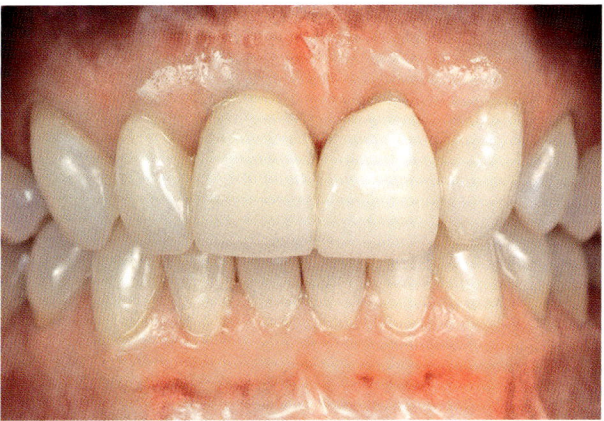

Fig 6-72 23 March 2007: anterior view in centric occlusion with visibility of the root apical to the finish line of the temporary crown on the left lateral incisor.

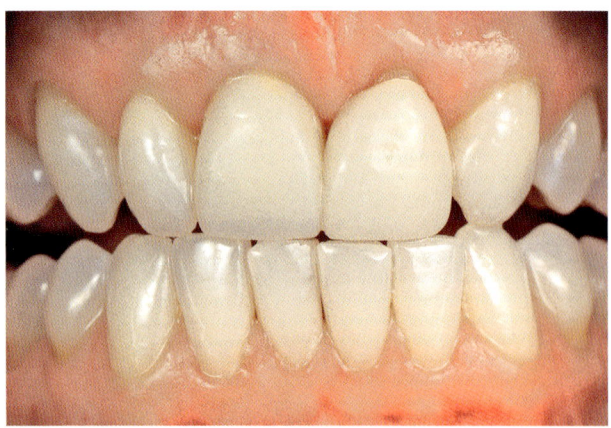

Fig 6-73 23 March 2007: anterior view in protrusion with visibility of the root apical to the finish line of the temporary crown on the left lateral incisor.

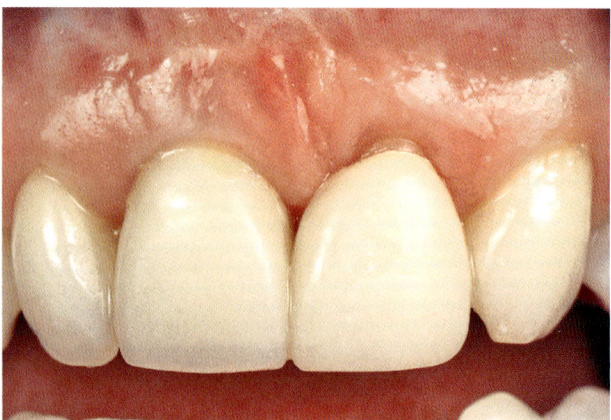

Fig 6-74 23 March 2007: anterior view showing visibility of the root apical to the finish line of the temporary crown on the left lateral incisor.

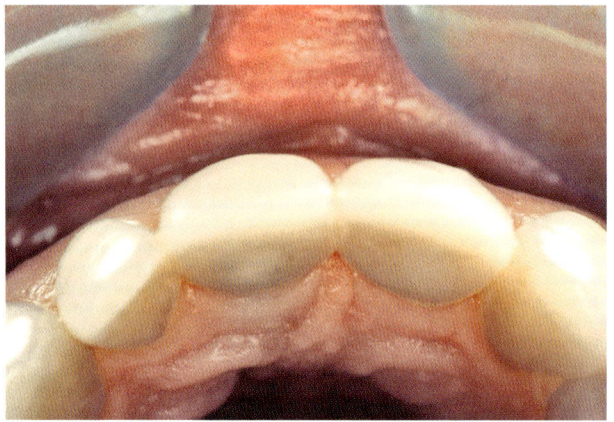

Fig 6-75 23 March 2007: incisal view of provisional crowns.

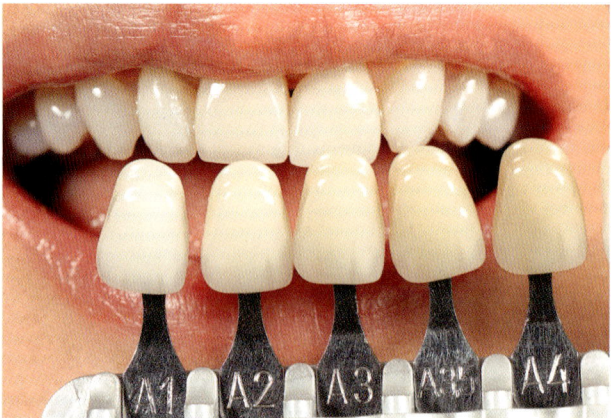

Fig 6-76 May 2007: shade analysis before home bleaching.

procedure for coronal repositioning of the FGM. The patient declined further surgery, and because the summer holidays were approaching, she wished to wait until September 2007, when impressions for the definitive crowns were planned, in the hope that the FGM might grow to a more coronal position. During this interim period, home bleaching was performed. Photographs were taken prebleaching (Fig 6-76) and postbleaching (September 2007) (Fig 6-77).

On 5 September 2007, the FGM around the left lateral incisor had crept to a more coronal position, and although it was not ideal, the patient decided to accept its location (Fig 6-78). The temporary crowns were removed and impressions for the definitive crowns made (Figs 6-79 to 6-81). Another waxup of the central incisors was carried out to visualize morphology, texture, and alignment for the definitive crowns (Fig 6-82). A zirconia abutment was

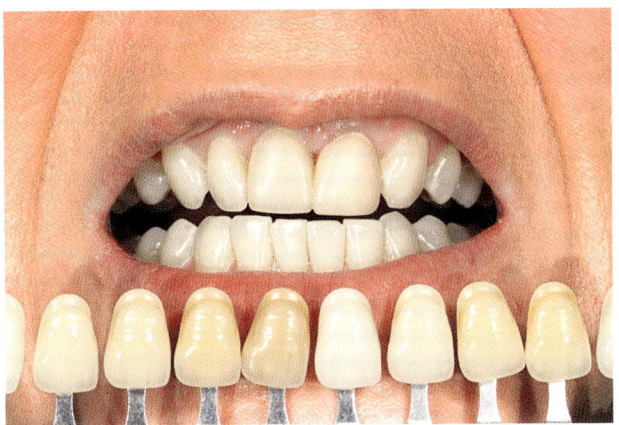

Fig 6-77 September 2007: shade analysis after home bleaching.

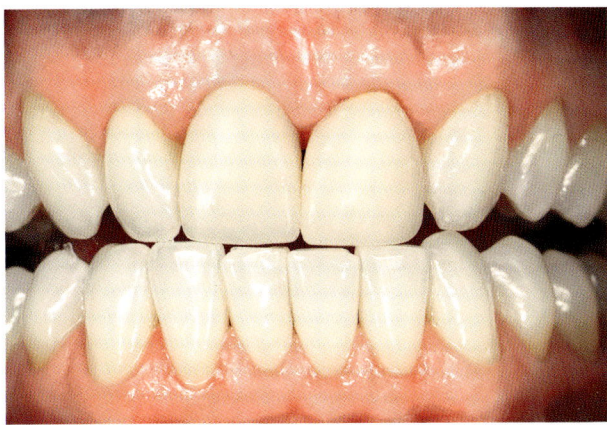

Fig 6-78 September 2007: anterior view. Notice that the FGM of the left lateral incisor has crept to a more coronal position.

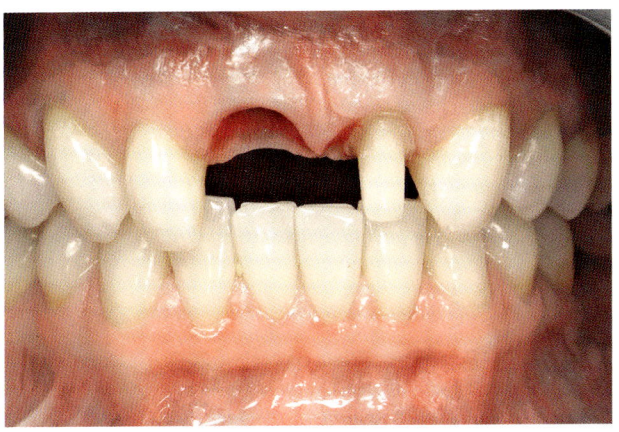

Fig 6-79 September 2007: anterior view showing removal of the provisional crowns for the definitive impressions.

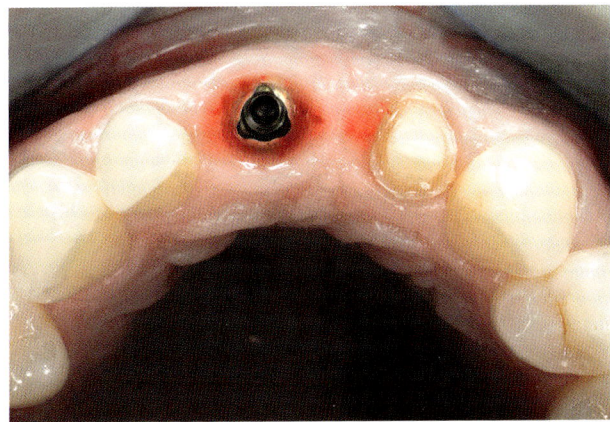

Fig 6-80 September 2007: incisal view showing removal of the provisional crowns for the definitive impressions.

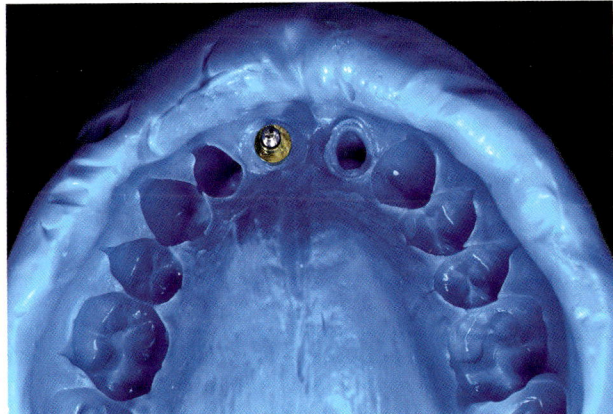

Fig 6-81 September 2007: impression at implant level using a coping and the prepared left lateral incisor.

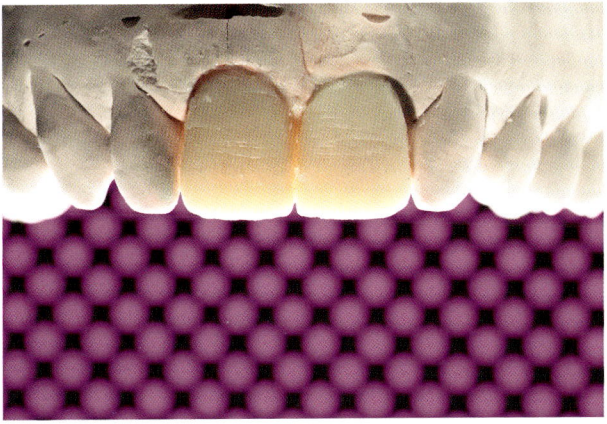

Fig 6-82 September 2007: diagnostic waxup of central incisors.

6 Vicissitudes of Two Maxillary Incisors Over 21 Years

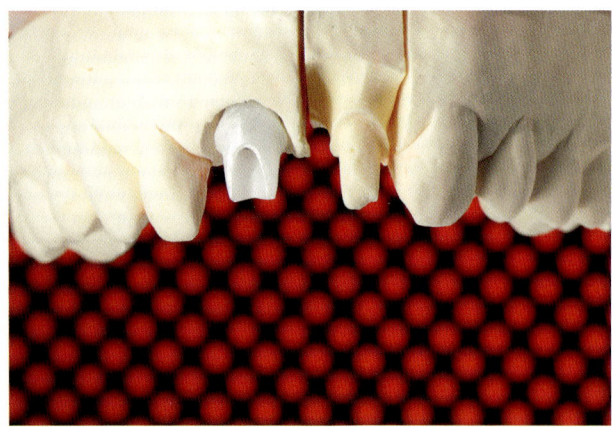

Fig 6-83 September 2007: anterior view of zirconia abutment for implant at the right central incisor site.

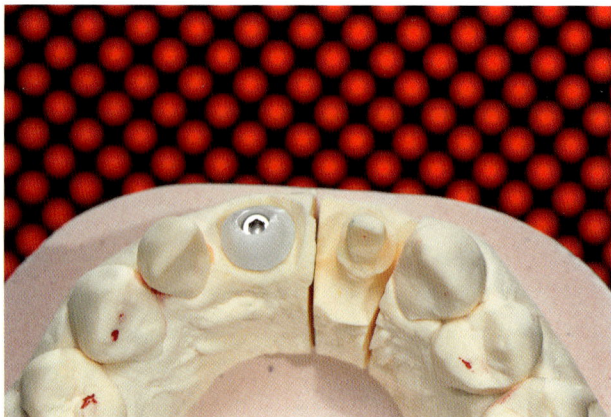

Fig 6-84 September 2007: incisal view of zirconia abutment for implant at the right central incisor site.

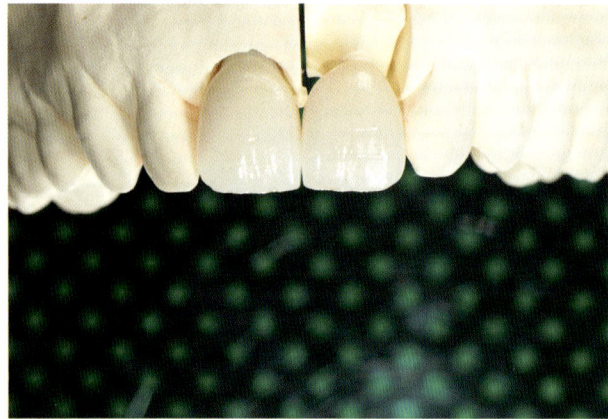

Fig 6-85 September 2007: anterior view of two completed Empress 2 crowns.

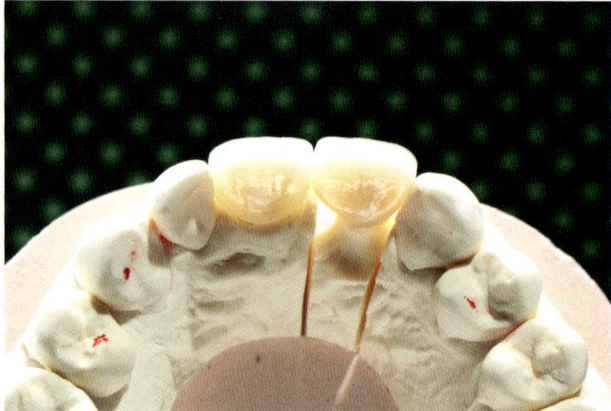

Fig 6-86 September 2007: incisal view of two completed Empress 2 crowns.

fabricated for the cement-retained crown to improve esthetics and to avoid shine through of a titanium abutment through the thin transmucosal tissues (Figs 6-83 and 6-84). Two Empress 2 crowns (Ivolcar-Vivadent, Liechtenstein) were fabricated for the central incisors (Figs 6-85 and 6-86).

First Try-in

Upon delivery of the crowns, the first try-in was carried out by placing the crowns on to the respective abutments (zirconia and natural tooth) (Figs 6-87 to 6-97). Esthetic scrutiny revealed that the shade, incisal translucency, and characterizations (such as calcification areas) blended impeccably with the adjacent dentition, but the following flaws required addressing.

6 Vicissitudes of Two Maxillary Incisors Over 21 Years

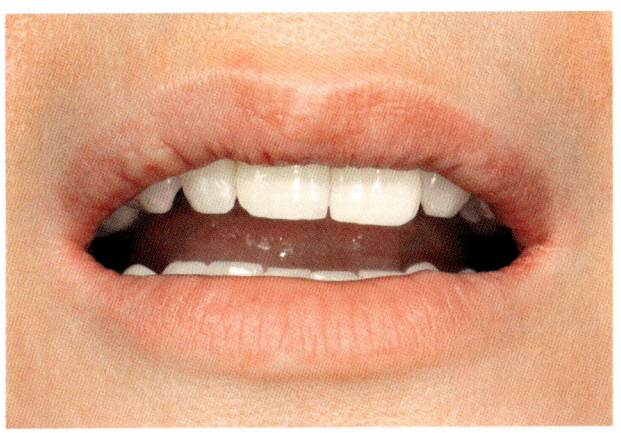

Fig 6-87 to 7-97 September, 2007: first try-in – see text for details.

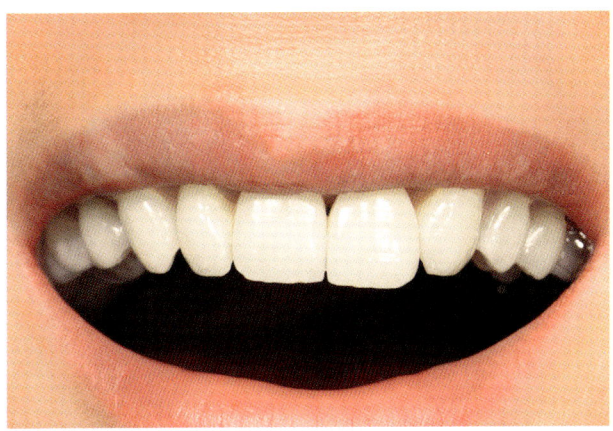

Fig 6-88

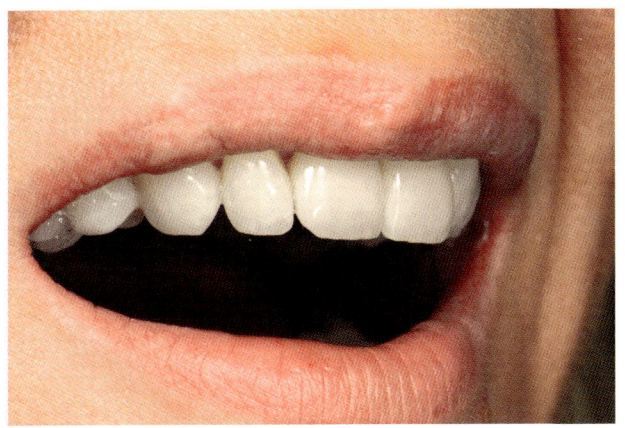

Fig 6-89

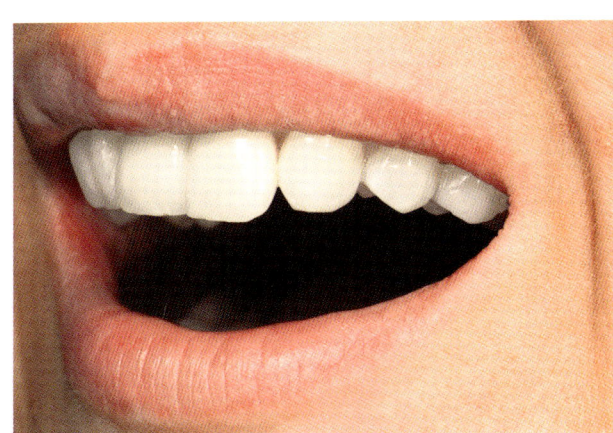

Fig 6-90

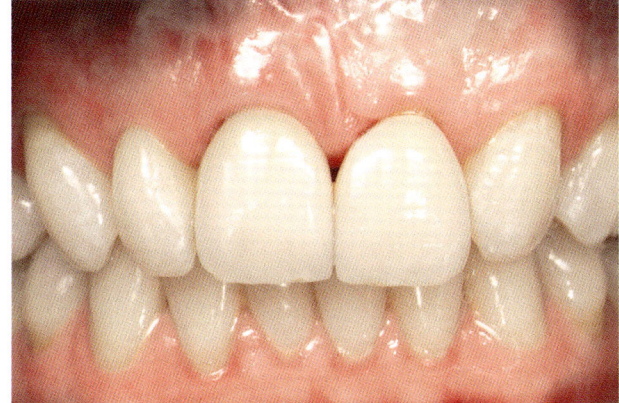

Fig 6-91

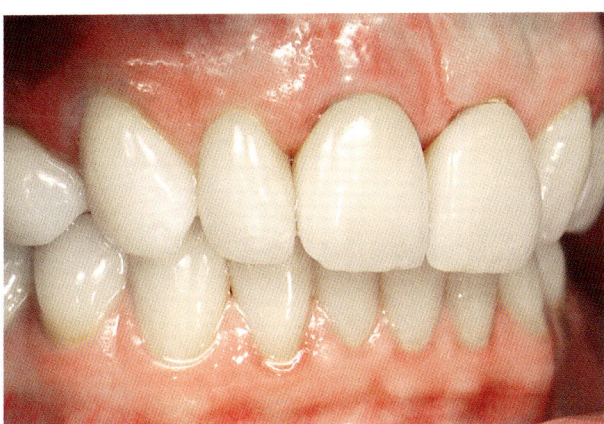

Fig 6-92

6 Vicissitudes of Two Maxillary Incisors Over 21 Years

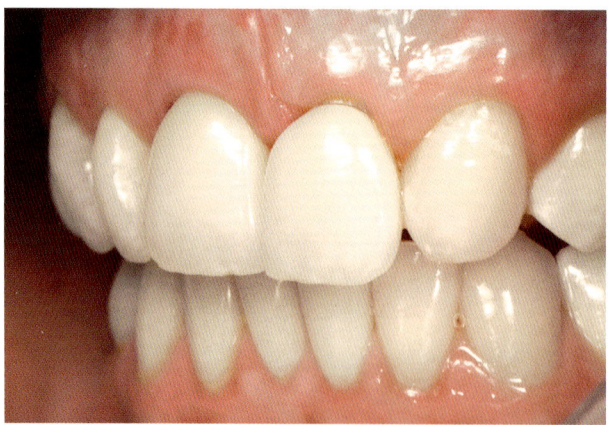
Fig 6-93

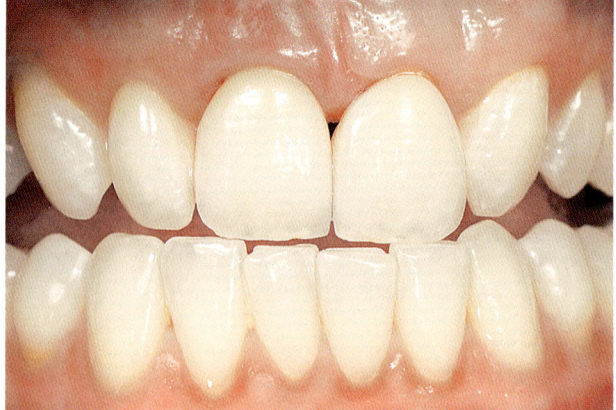
Fig 6-94

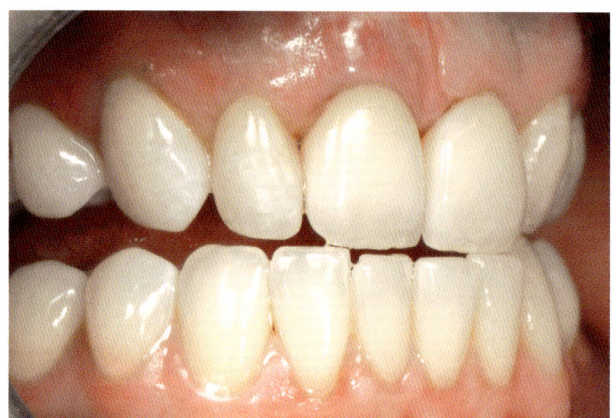
Fig 6-95

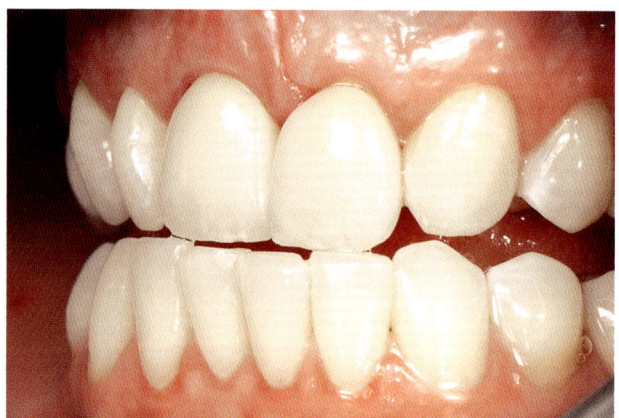
Fig 6-96

- The distal embrasure of the right central incisor was rounded, requiring a sharper line angle to create a squarer tooth (see Figs 6-87 to 6-89, 6-91, 6-92, 6-94, 6-95).
- left lateral incisor (simulating a central incisor) was the main concern, with the following flaws.
  - The buccal crown margin was open (Figs 6-91 to 6-96).
  - The mesial and distal contours on the facial aspect were bulbous compared with the right central (Fig 6-97).
  - The tooth appeared longer than the right central incisor (Figs 6-87 to 6-96), which resulted in initial contact during protrusion with the mandibular teeth, while a space was evident between the right central and lower incisors (Figs 6-94 to 6-96).

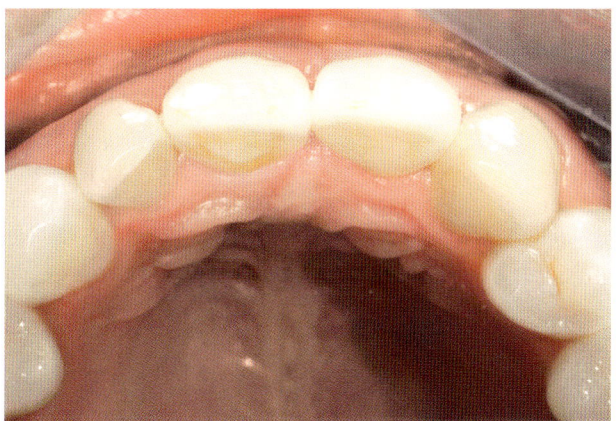
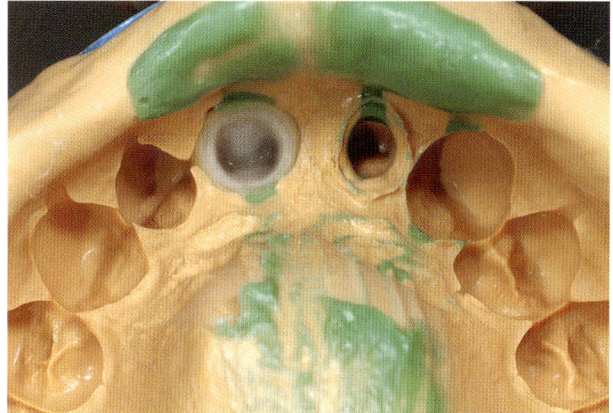

Fig 6-97

Fig 6-98 September, 2007: impression to rectify the deficient cervical crown margin on the left crown.

- The central incisors were not mirror images. This was a difficult task to achieve because the abutment preparations were of different teeth (a central and a lateral incisor). In addition, because the left canine was adjacent to the simulated left central incisor, the incisal embrasure was exaggerated and, therefore, different from that on the right side. This disparity was difficult to address unless the left canine was also provided with a crown to simulate a lateral incisor.
- There was a median maxillary "black triangle", which could be resolved by moving the contact point more apically (Fig 6-94). However, this procedure often compromises the mesial contours, resulting in oddly shaped crowns.
- During protrusion, the palatal aspect of the crown was contacting the lower teeth more than the right central crown. The aberrant contact was judicially removed until contact was uniform on both crowns.

To resolve the deficient margin on the buccal aspect of the left crown, the right crown was left in situ, retraction cord was placed around the left lateral incisor to visualize the preparation finish lines, and a new impression was made, picking-up the right crown (Fig 6-98).

Second Try-In

The necessary modifications were carried out in the dental laboratory, and the crowns were returned for a second try-in on 29 October 2007. The deficient buccal margin on the left crown was rectified. The length and bulbosity were also reduced, but not enough to satisfy the patient (Figs 6-99 and 6-100). Photographs were taken and the crowns marked with a pencil to indicate further alterations (ie, bulbosity and length), and the crowns were returned to the ceramist. The adjustments could have been performed chairside, but there

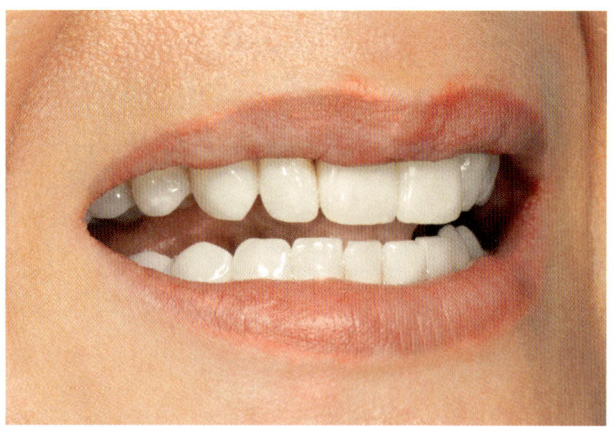
Fig 6-99 October 2007: second try-in – see text for details.

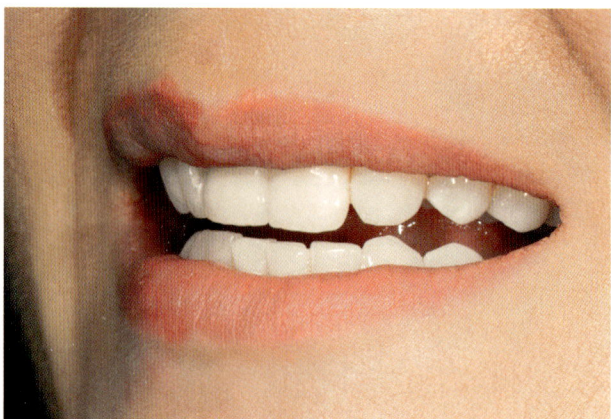
Fig 6-100 October 2007: second try-in.

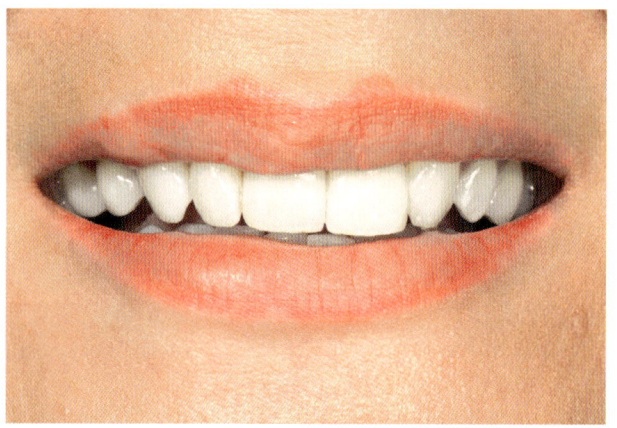
Fig 6-101 November 2007: third try-in – see text for details.

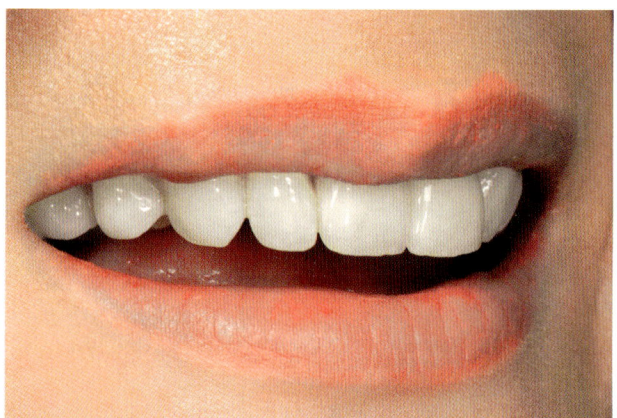
Fig 6-102 November 2007: third try-in.

is always the possibility of fracturing the veneering porcelain. Furthermore, reglazing in a furnace is essential to seal surface flaws of any ceramic material following alterations.

Third Try-in

At the third try-in, on 14 November 2007, the patient was still unhappy. Although she accepted there were improvements on the second try-in, her comments were as follows (Figs 6-101 to 6-103).

- She felt that the crowns were not mirror images.
- She preferred the general appearance of the crowns at the second try-in but could not articulate the reasons why.

6 Vicissitudes of Two Maxillary Incisors Over 21 Years

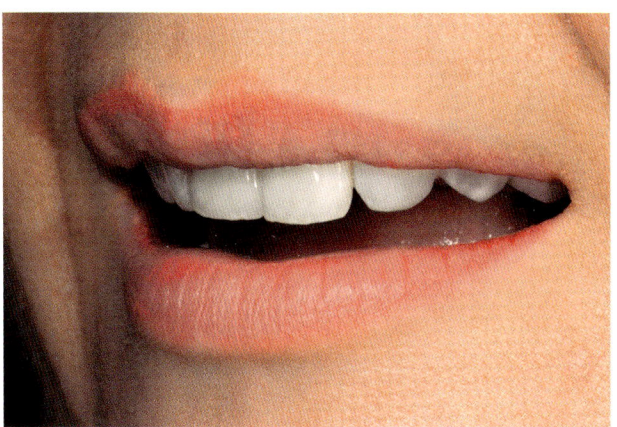

Fig 6-103 November 2007: third try-in.

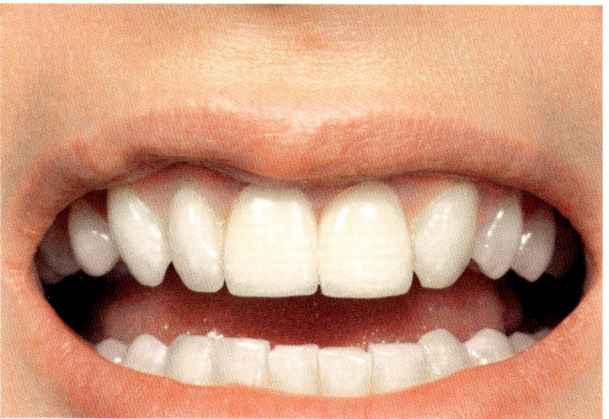

Fig 6-104 December 2007: fourth try-in – see text for details.

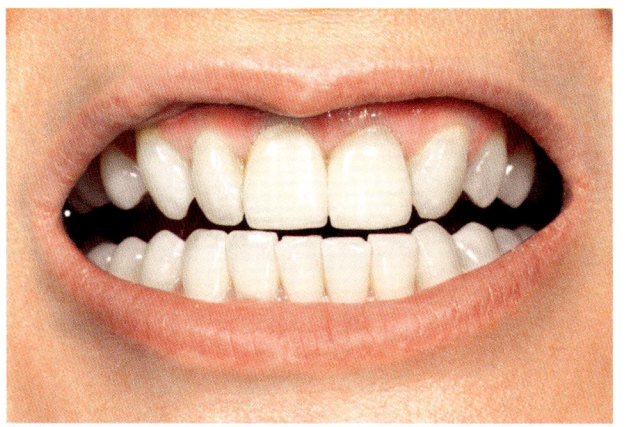

Fig 6-105 December 2007: fourth try-in.

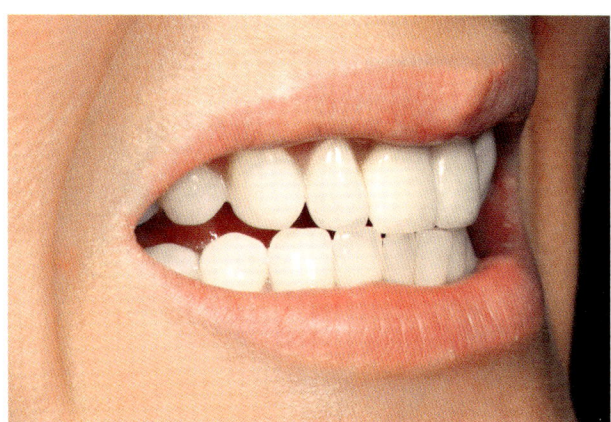

Fig 6-106 December 2007: fourth try-in.

Fourth Try-in

At this stage, the ceramist who had attempted to resolve the esthetic anomalies and satisfy the patient for the preceding three try-ins felt he could do no more. He came to the conclusion that despite his efforts, he was unable to satisfy the patient's wishes.

On 29 November 2007, impressions were taken and forwarded to another ceramist, who fabricated two IPS e.max crowns (Ivoclar-Vivadent, Liechtenstein) and a try-in was scheduled for 10 December 2007 (Figs 6-104 to 6-107). The analysis was as follows.

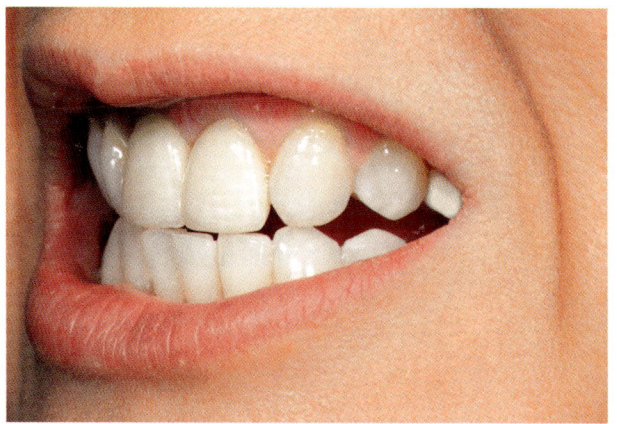

Fig 6-107 December 2007: fourth try-in.

89

6 Vicissitudes of Two Maxillary Incisors Over 21 Years

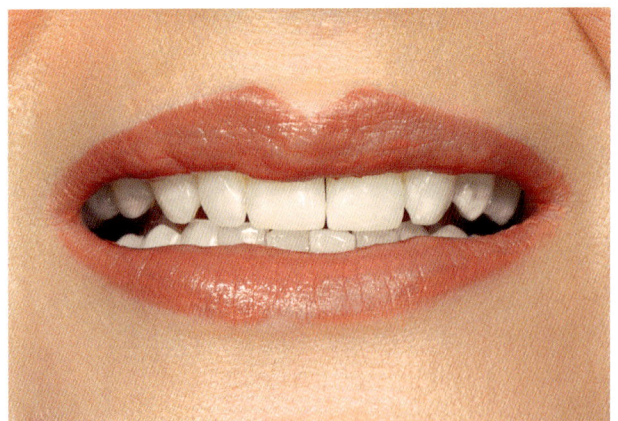

Fig 6-108 January 2008: postoperative result.

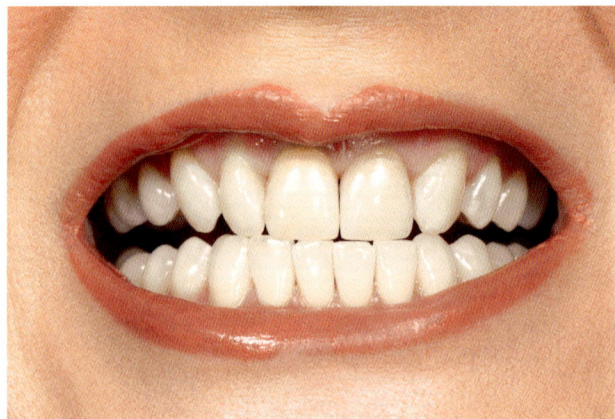

Fig 6-109 January 2008: postoperative result.

- The patient was happy with the shapes of both crowns.
- A pseudo-pontic was created on the mesial aspect of the left crown to close the gingival embrasure.
- Both crowns were too opaque, requiring more translucency to blend with the surrounding natural teeth.
- The incisal one third of the crowns were too protrusive, requiring a more palatal inclination (see Fig 6-106).

The crowns were returned for further adjustments, and an appointment made for the new year.

Postoperative result

On 7 January 2008, the ceramist had carried out the necessary amendments and the patient was satisfied with the result (Figs 6-108 to 6-113). The intaglio surface of the left crown was treated with hydrofluoric acid and silane, and the tooth abutment with a dentine-bonding agent (iBond, Heraeus, Hanau, Germany); the crown was luted with a resin-based cement (Variolink II, Ivoclar-Vivadent, Liechtenstein). The crown on the right was supported by a zirconia abutment and luted with TempBond (KerrHawe, Switzerland).

It is interesting to notice that after four try-ins, what the patient really wanted was that the crowns should be a similar shape to her original PLVs (compare Fig 6-25 with 6-108). The previous ceramist have strived to create more natural oval-shaped crowns, with subtle chips and staining at the incisal edges (see Fig 6-88), which the patient rejected in favor of a squarer shape and sharper line angles (see Fig 6-110). This demonstrates two points. The first is that a communication breakdown between patient, dentist, and ceramist can be a major cause of problems. Second, in esthetic dentistry, the ceramist and dentist should not impose their wishes on to patients. Patient

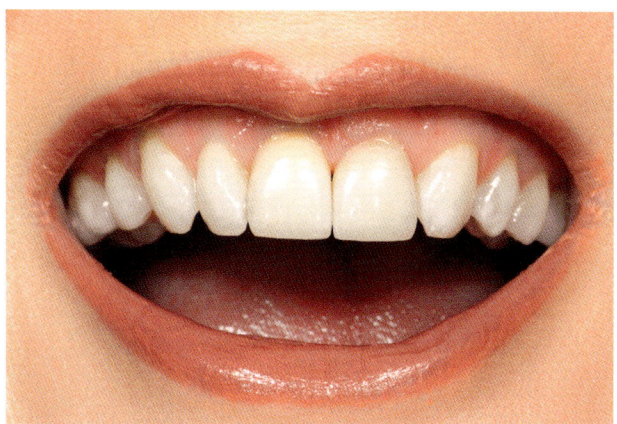
Fig 6-110 January 2008: postoperative result.

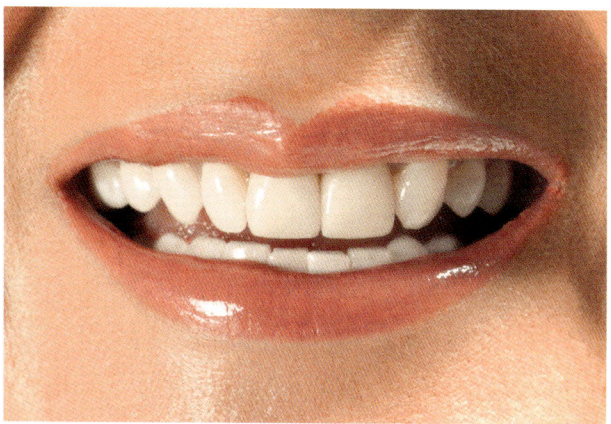
Fig 6-111 January 2008: postoperative result.

involvement is essential at the outset, along with the presumption that their wishes take precedence (assuming that clinical feasibility is not compromised) over those of all other protagonists in the dental team. The final result is esthetically debatable and many will disagree with the patient's decision, preferring the crowns at previous try-in stages. However, the patient is the final arbiter.

Discussion

The accident that avulsed the patient's left central incisor was, of course, unfortunate. But the ensuing poor dental treatment added to the failing fortunes of the right central incisor. It is probable that the impact also devitalized the right central incisor. However, the tooth was not root filled at the time of the initial treatment, which allowed accumulation and proliferation of bacteria in the root canal and apical regions. Although root fillings were subsequently attempted (with limited success), the prognosis of the tooth was placed in jeopardy at the onset. Furthermore, the subsequent veneers on the right central and, later, on the left lateral incisors were also defective, which compounded the bacterial insult through plaque accumulation. However, it is important to realize that, PLVs were a relatively novel modality in 1986. Although PLVs were conceived many decades earlier, their use in general practice was not widespread. There was ambiguity about whether tooth preparation was necessary before providing a PLV. If no preparation was carried out, the final veneer would appear bulbous, while aggressive tooth preparation exposed dentin, and dentin-bonding agents at the time were not as efficacious as they are today. Another compromise was that the benefits of immediate dentin sealing following tooth preparation was unknown and not widely practiced, which added to dentin contamination. Also, adhesive dentistry was in its infancy, and techniques were

6 Vicissitudes of Two Maxillary Incisors Over 21 Years

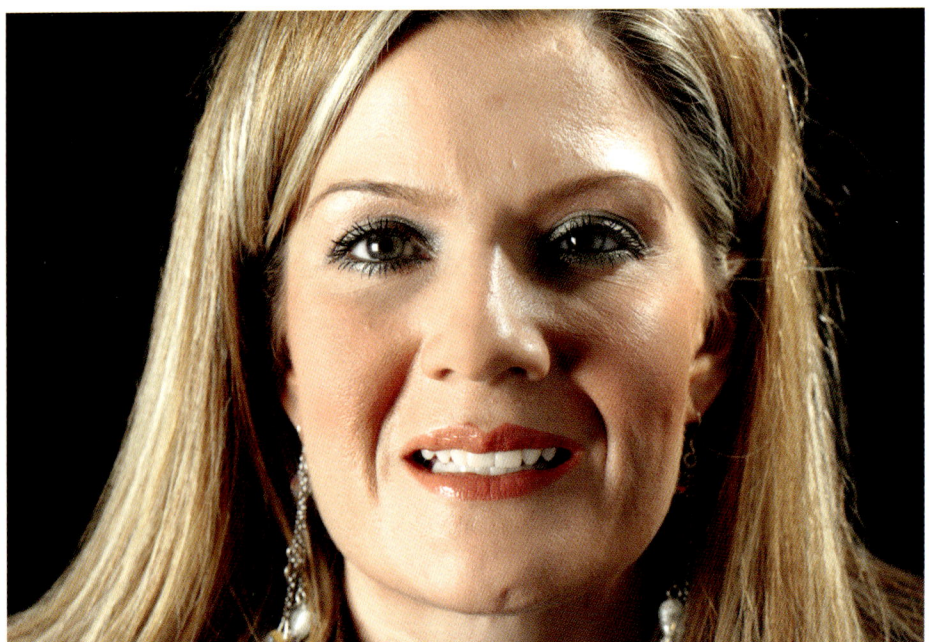

Fig 6-112 January 2008: postoperative result.

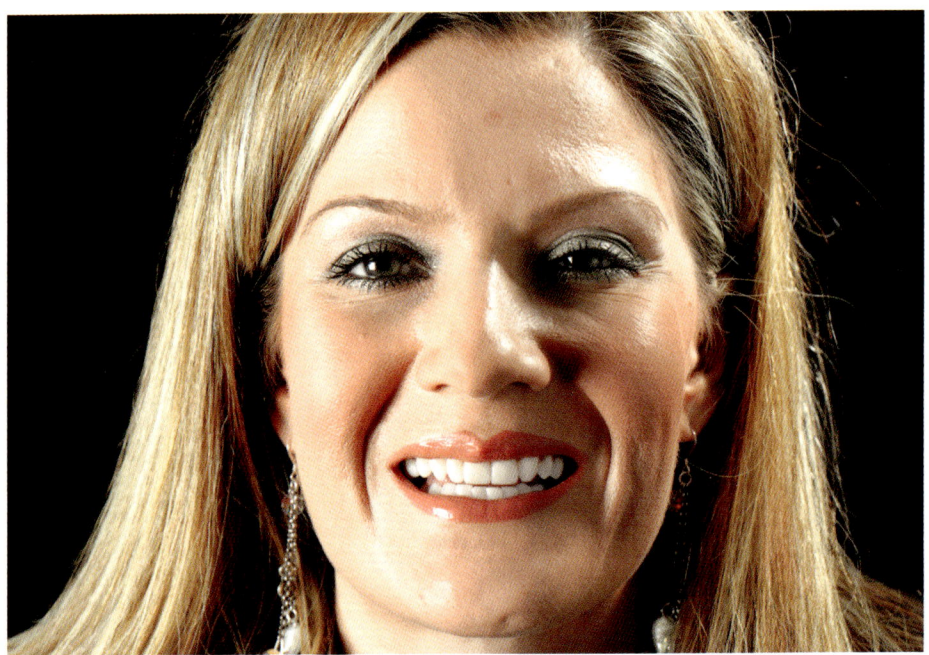

Fig 6-113 January 2008: postoperative result.

relatively archaic compared with current standards. Therefore, given the circumstances, the treatment provided was the best available at that time.

The turning point in this case study, and a crucial decision for the patient, was whether or not to extract the right central incisor. Although the initial apicectomy allowed the tooth to survive for nearly a decade, it was not without problems. There were several sporadic episodes of acute infection, which required antibiotic intervention, time off work, and undue pain, suffering, and anxiety. In addition, the root discoloration was an esthetic concern, which could have been mitigated by nonvital bleaching had the patient decided to pursue another apicectomy.

There are two main negative aspects of repeating an apicectomy. First, the shortening of the root may result in an unfavorable root to crown ratio, creating instability of the crown and mobility of the tooth. Second, the apical site would be subjected to further surgical trauma, and so if any residual bacteria remained, the site would continue to be progressively compromised. As a result, extensive augmentation would be required if an implant were to be considered at a later date. Augmentation is not an impossible task, but considering the location of this tooth, soft and hard tissue grafting would be challenging and unpredictable for achieving superlative esthetics. This fact is clearly highlighted by the crown lengthening on the left lateral incisor, as soft tissue healing is unpredictable, often yielding unsatisfactory and capricious outcomes.

The discussion above about providing PLVs in 1986 is also applicable to current implant therapy. However, as science advances, techniques become refined, and the understanding of biological principles is enhanced, the protocols currently adopted for implants may become redundant, or even frowned upon, in 21 years' time.

Another aspect of this case study is the emphasis on the need for patient participation in esthetic dentistry. Esthetics, unlike irrefutable scientific principles, is fraught with subjectivity. At the first try-in, the open margin, of course, needed to be rectified. However, most of the esthetic flaws identified in the subsequent try-ins are questionable, but nevertheless they are a concern. Even if treatment satisfies all scientific criteria, it may still be judged a failure by the patient; as esthetic dental practitioners, it is our obligation to satisfy not only scientific criteria but also the person we are treating. At times, this can be frustrating and onerous, but as clinicians we should be conduits, not judges, for our patients' desires.

The ultimate aim of this case study is to show that failures can, and do, happen. The most effective method of managing failure is to acknowledge it, rectify it, and learn from it. Success is the result of learning from failure, not ignoring it, and experience is gained from consternation, rarely from satisfaction.

Restitution of Anterior Dental Esthetics with a Variety of Restorations

Ceramics by Willi Geller, Zurich, Switzerland

Pre- and Postoperative Status

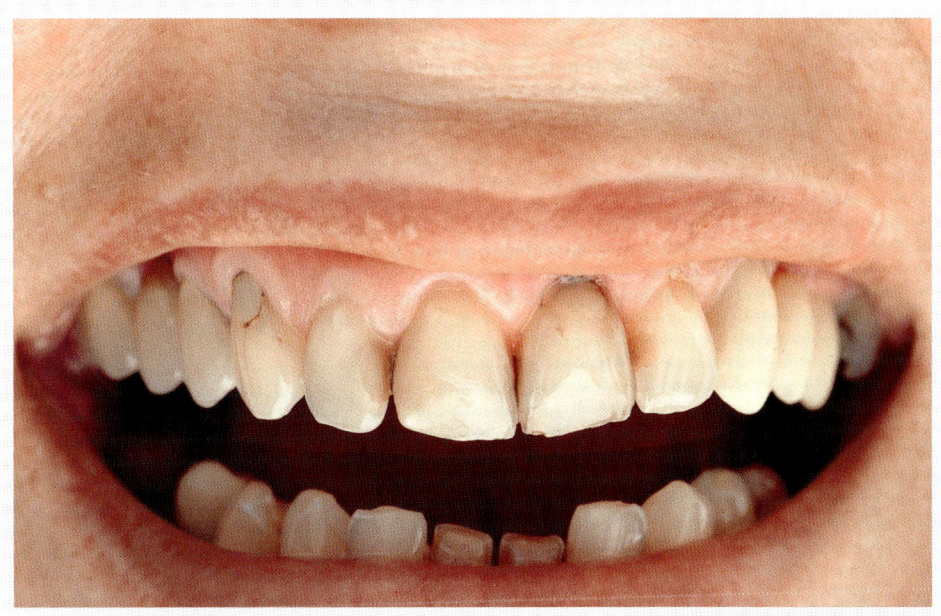

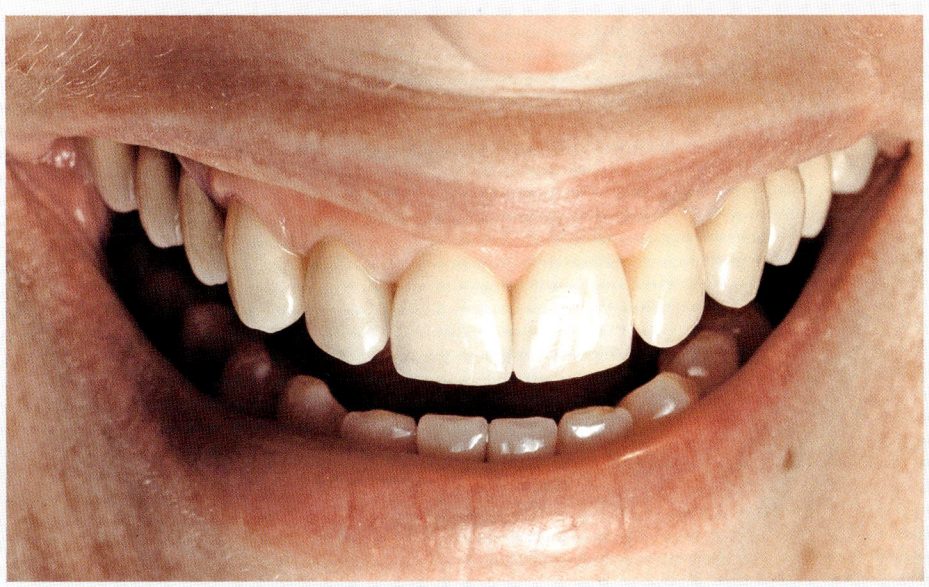

Dental History

Most of the dental history of this patient, a 56-year-old woman, revolved around poor-quality dentistry combined with tooth wear from abrasion and erosion of the mandibular incisors caused by lemon sucking. Her desire was to enhance her smile, prevent further deterioration, and safeguard her dentition.

Preoperative Status

The periodontal health was poor, exacerbated by defective restorations, which were causing plaque accumulation. There were innumerable resin-composite fillings, which had been repeatedly replaced over many decades. Combined with this poor dentistry was toothbrush abrasion and acidic erosion. All these factors contributed to an abnormal anatomical tooth form, an uneven or "roller-coaster" incisal plane, tooth discoloration, and gingival embrasures or "black triangles". Also, the metal-ceramic fixed partial denture (FPD) from the maxillary left canine to the second premolar had grossly open margins, acting as a niche for bacteria and an annoying food trap (Figs 7-1 and 7-2).

Treatment Options

1. Achieve periodontal health and assess endodontic status prior to considering any of the following options.
2. Bleach teeth and replace the resin-composite fillings and the defective FPD.
3. Place indirect restorations to restore health (periodontal and endodontic), function (occlusion and phonetics), and esthetics (form, color, and incisal plane), conforming to the HFA triad (health, function, and aesthetics).

Scientific Credence for Treatment Options

This case study demonstrates two key aspects of dental care. The first is sequentially achieving health, function, and esthetics, and the second is choosing the most appropriate type and material of a restoration.

The first stage is to restore the health of the periodontium by prophylaxis and then to review the endodontic status. Although the central incisors were heavily restored, radiographs revealed no apical pathology on any of the teeth. The occlusion was satisfactory, without interferences, and the temporomandibular joint was symptomless. Speech was slightly affected by air escaping between the upper and lower anterior incisors, especially during "s" sounds.

Bleaching the maxillary and mandibular teeth would resolve discoloration, but not the morphology or the erratic incisal plane. Resin-composite fillings would be an acceptable option, but since these had been repeatedly replaced, the structural integrity of some teeth, especially the maxillary central incisors, was severely compromised.

7 Restitution of Anterior Dental Esthetics with a Variety of Restorations

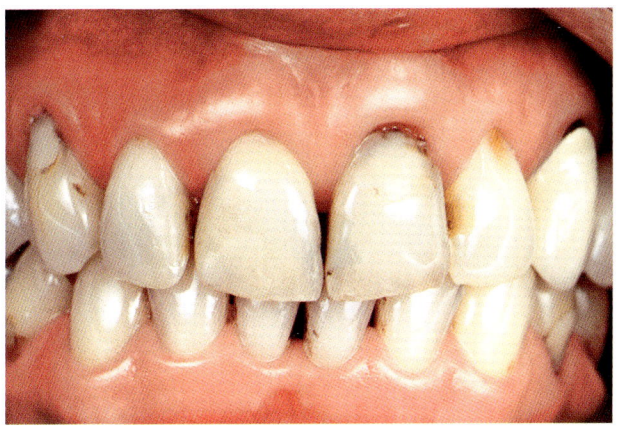

Fig 7-1 Preoperative anterior view.

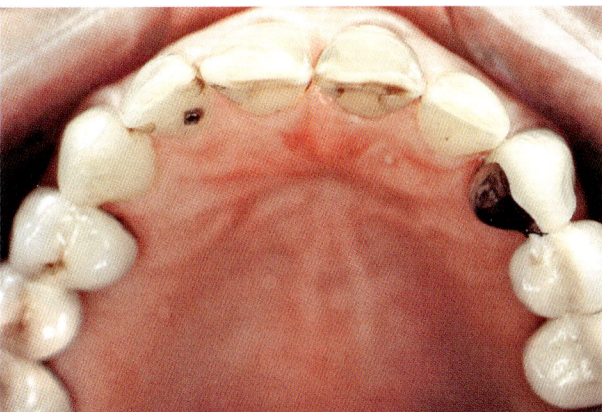

Fig 7-2 Preoperative incisal view.

Indirect restorations would be more invasive, but have the advantage of achieving many of the treatment objectives (ie, color, form, and rebuilding the maxillary incisal plane).

Clinical Erudition and Feasibility

Bleaching teeth, replacing resin-composite fillings, and achieving periodontal health are all relatively straightforward. However, if indirect restorations are the chosen option, correct decision-making regarding type of restoration, choice of materials, etc. is essential for a favorable and long-lasting outcome. A systematic approach to adopt when choosing a restoration is to consider:
1. type of restoration
2. material(s) for the restoration
3. margin location of the restoration.

The scheme in Box 7-1 (see next page) summarizes the guidelines on the choice of restorations. Finally, for an indirect restoration option, a skilled ceramist is required to integrate and blend the shade of the different types of restoration and material with the natural dentition.

Patient Needs and Wants

The bleaching option was attractive as it was the least invasive, but bleaching would not resolve all the prevailing esthetic anomalies. Furthermore, the patient was reticent about replacing the existing resin-composite fillings with similar ones owing to her poor experience with previous direct restorations. She wished to pursue the indirect option for superlative esthetics.

97

Box 7-1 Guidelines for the choice of restorations.

1. Type of restoration
    a. Direct – preferable where possible, minimally invasive.
    b. Indirect:
        i. Partial coverage – for minimum color and shape changes.
        ii. Full coverage – indicted for the following reasons:
            1. Existing full-coverage restoration(s).
            2. Compromised structural integrity – eg, palatal erosion, extensive fillings or fractures.
            3. Changing occlusal vertical dimension.
            4. High-strength materials required for FPDs – eg, alumina or zirconia.
            5. Pronounced color change.
            6. Pronounced misalignment, where orthodontics are contraindicated or refused.

2. Choice of material
    Ascertain what requires replacing: enamel, or enamel and dentin?
    a. Direct – resin-composite fillings with dentin-bonding agents.
    b. Indirect:
        i. Metal or metal-ceramic – indicted for the following reasons:
            1. FPDs.
            2. Occlusion – eg, for steep anterior guidance or bruxism.
            3. Discoloration – eg, to mask pronounced discoloration or metal cores.
        ii. Ceramics – indicted for strength and esthetics:
            1. Strength – alumina or zirconia (for FPDs, bruxism, steep anterior guidance).
            2. Discoloration – eg, lithium disilicate, alumina, or zirconia (to mask discoloration).
            3. Esthetics – eg, feldspathic, leucite glass (with acceptable color of underlying tooth substrate), or lithium disilicate.

3. Margin location
    a. Low lip line – supragingival.
    b. High lip line – equigingival or subgingival:
        i. Color change.
        ii. Discolored underlying substrate.
        iii. Using less-translucent (dense) materials – eg, zirconia.
        iv. Periodontal biotype – thick (subgingival), thin (supragingival).
    c. Break contact points – color and shape change.
    d. Incisal coverage – increase length or alter shape.

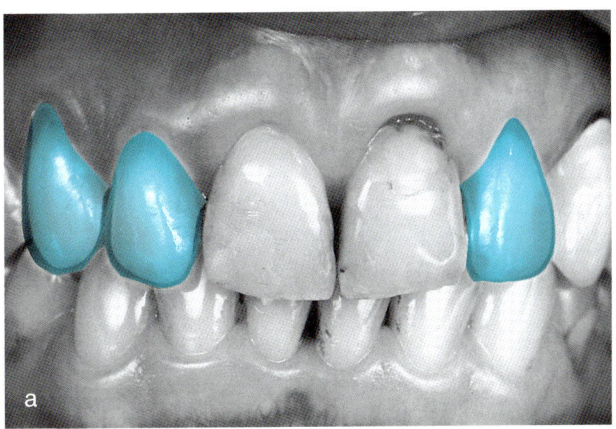 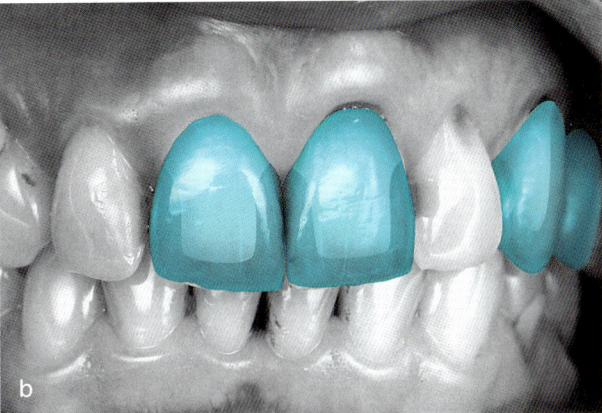

Fig 7-3 Types of restoration chosen: (a) partial coverage, (b) full coverage.

Treatment Sequence

Treatment was required on the maxillary canines and incisors, the existing three-unit FPD (from the maxillary left canine to the second premolar), and the mandibular central incisors. Using the above scheme, decisions were made regarding the type of restoration, the materials, and the margin location.

Type of Restoration

For the maxillary lateral incisors and right canine and the mandibular central incisors, porcelain laminate veneers (PLVs) were the ideal choice. The rationale was that only minimal color and shape changes were necessary, and limiting coverage to the facial aspect would keep the remaining tooth intact (Fig 7-3a).

Full coverage was indicated for the maxillary central incisors owing to the existing large resin-composite fillings, which extended palatally (Fig 7-3b). Furthermore, after removing the old fillings and any decay, the structural integrity of these teeth would be compromised, warranting extracoronal prostheses. The existing three-unit FPD obviously had to be replaced with a new FPD (Fig 7-3b).

Choice of Material

Since esthetics were a paramount concern, and in the absence of occlusal problems, silica ceramics were the best choice for the PLVs and the full-coverage crowns. Silica ceramics are relatively weak, but they have a high glass content with increased translucency, allowing the underlying tooth substrate to shine through and so give depth and a life-like appearance to a restoration. Choices of silica materials include feldspathic porcelain (fabricated on platinum foil or refractory dies), leucite glass (Empress 1, Ivolcar-Vivadent, Lichtenstein), or lithium disilicate (Empress 2). In this case, unilayer feldspathic porcelain, fabricated on platinum foil, was chosen to keep tooth preparation to a minimum (Fig 7-4a). For bilayer restorations, such as Empress 1 and 2,

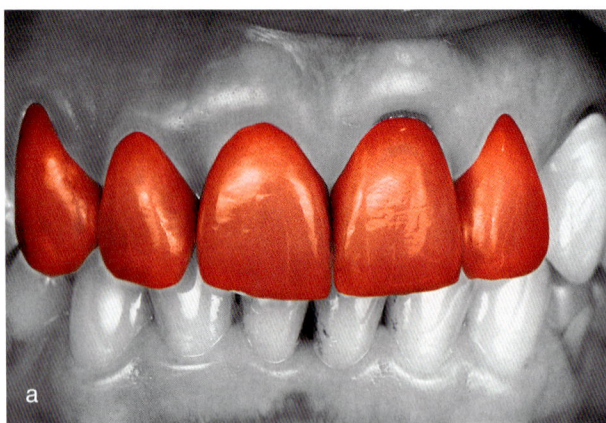 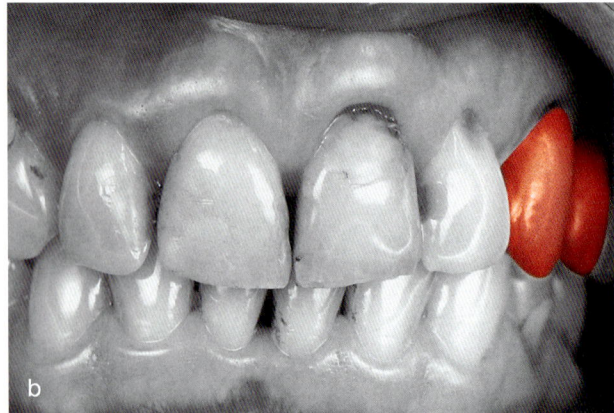

Fig 7-4 Types of material chosen: (a) feldspathic porcelain, (b) metal-ceramic.

additional tooth reduction is necessary to accommodate the coping or substructure. However, if the underlying tooth is discolored and requires masking, a bilayer system, such as Empress 2 (Ivolcar-Vivadent, Liechtenstein) or Procera (Nobel Biocare, Sweden), is an option worth considering.

FPDs can be fabricated using either metal-ceramics or high-strength ceramics such as zirconia. The former was chosen simply for the reason of long-term clinical success (Fig 7-4b). Zirconia is a promising material, but data on long-term performance or clinical trails regarding posterior FPDs are sparse.

Margin Location

The patient has a moderately high lip line and a thick biotype, which are favorable for a subgingival margin location for all the restoration (Fig 7-5a). The proximal contacts were broken (Fig 7-5b) to harmonize the shades of the veneering porcelain of three different types of restorations (PLVs, full-coverage all-ceramic crowns, and a metal-ceramic FPD). Finally, to restore the uneven incisal plane, incisal coverage was necessary for all PLV preparations (Fig 7-5c).

Treatment

Having chosen the types of restoration, restorative materials, and location of the margins, treatment was initiated by prophylaxis to improve periodontal health (Figs 7-6 and 7-7). One week later, tooth preparations for the PLVs were carried out on the maxillary right canine, right lateral incisor, and left lateral incisor, and on the mandibular central incisors. Preparations were also carried out for the full-coverage crowns on the maxillary central incisors. The FPD on the maxillary left canine and second premolar was removed, and the tooth preparations refined. Once gingival health was apparent after 1 week of temporization (Figs 7-8 and 7-9), impressions were attempted. The impressions recorded an area apical to the finish line, allowing the ceramist to create the

7 Restitution of Anterior Dental Esthetics with a Variety of Restorations

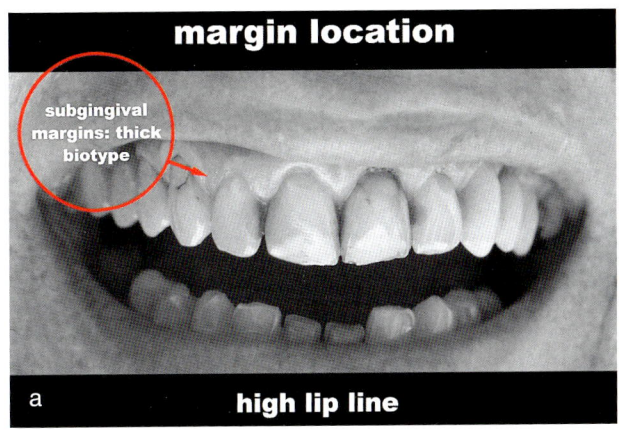

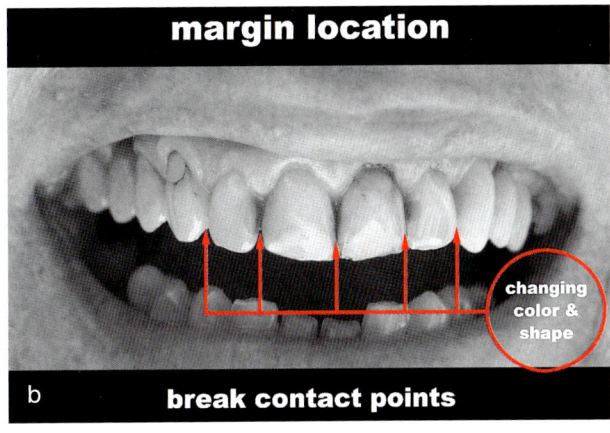

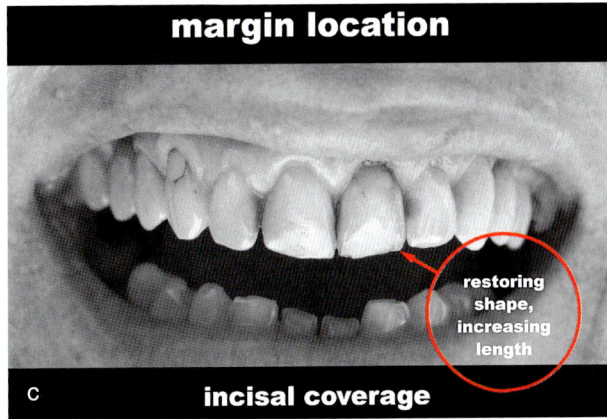

Fig 7-5 Margin location:
(a) subgingival margin location,
(b) broken proximal contacts,
(c) incisal coverage.

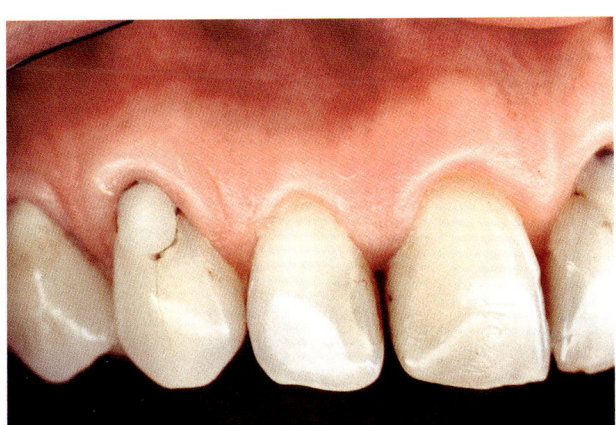

Fig 7-6 Right lateral view following prophylaxis.

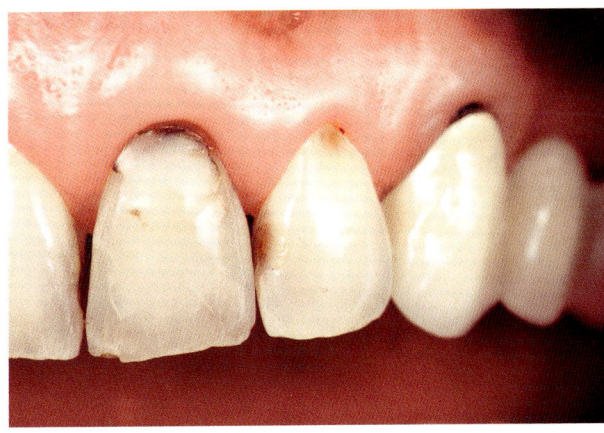

Fig 7-7 Left lateral view following prophylaxis.

7 Restitution of Anterior Dental Esthetics with a Variety of Restorations

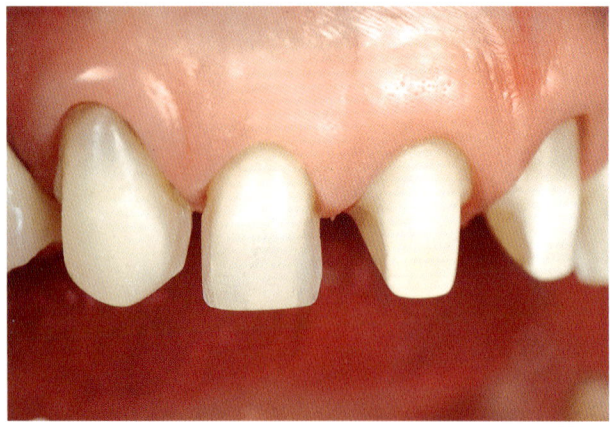

Fig 7-8 Right lateral view of tooth preparations, showing impeccable gingival health.

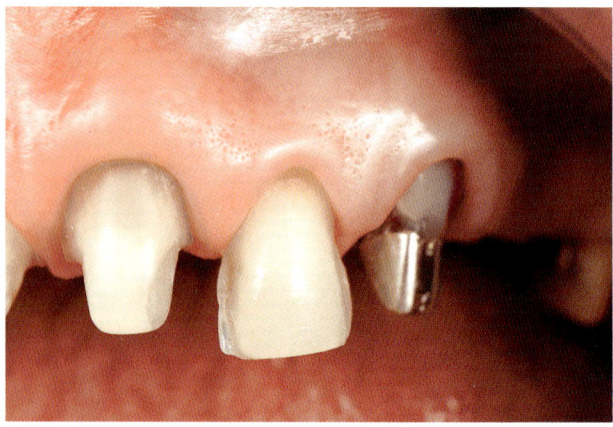

Fig 7-9 Left lateral view of tooth preparations, showing impeccable gingival health.

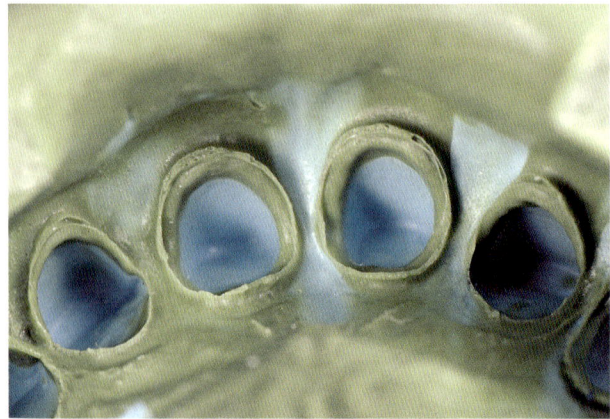

Fig 7-10 Impression of tooth preparations. Notice that an area apical to the finish line is faithfully recorded.

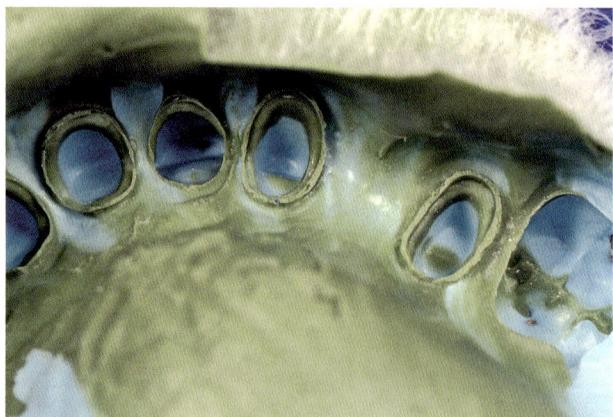

Fig 7-11 Impression of tooth preparations. Notice that an area apical to the finish line is faithfully recorded.

correct emergence profiles (Figs 7-10 and 7-11). After trimming the plaster model (Fig 7-12), the metal framework for the FPD was cast and cut back at the cervical margins (Fig 7-13). This allowed for a 360-degree porcelain shoulder for improved light transmission at the critical junction between restoration and teeth, and avoided the classic cervical shadowing, which is detrimental to esthetic appraisal. The completed restorations are shown in Figure 7-14, while Figures 7-15 and 7-16 show the relationship between the tooth preparations and the contours of the prostheses. Notice the correction of the roller-coaster incisal plane, which has been restored to a seamless concavity, parallel to the curvature of the mandibular lip during a relaxed smile (Fig 7-17).

The pre- and postoperative images (Figs 7-18 to 7-28) demonstrate the following outcomes.

7 Restitution of Anterior Dental Esthetics with a Variety of Restorations

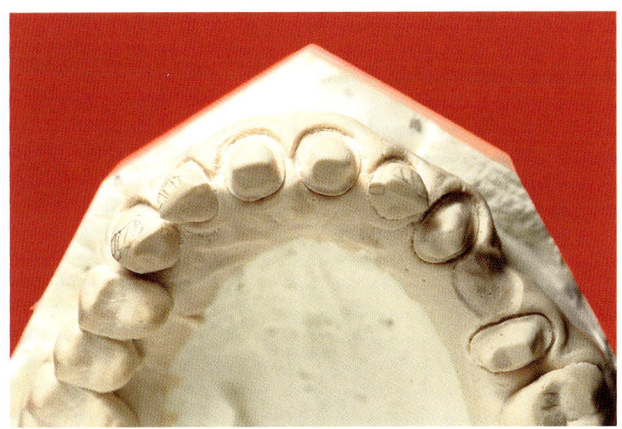

Fig 7-12 Plaster cast of tooth preparations.

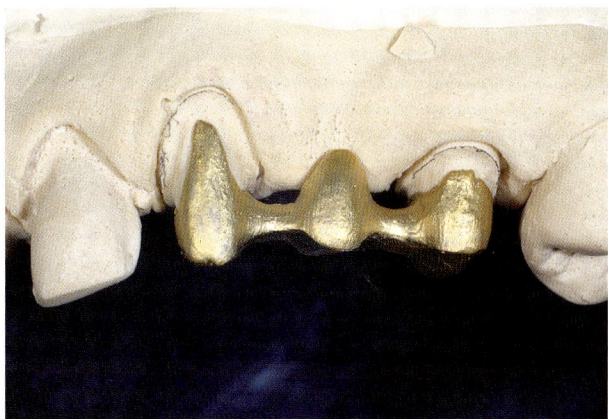

Fig 7-13 Metal cutback for ceramic shoulders on the metal-ceramic three-unit FPD.

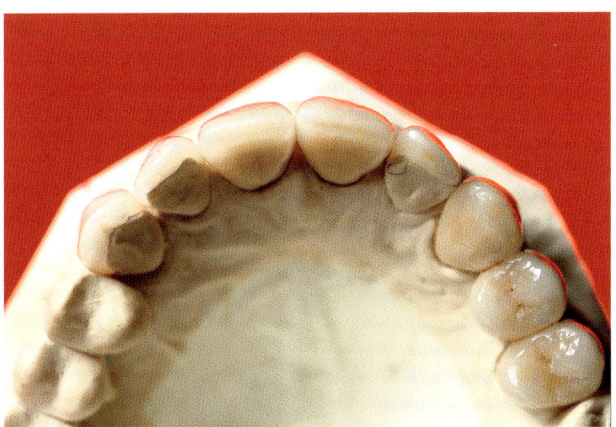

Fig 7-14 Completed definitive restorations on the plaster cast: incisal view.

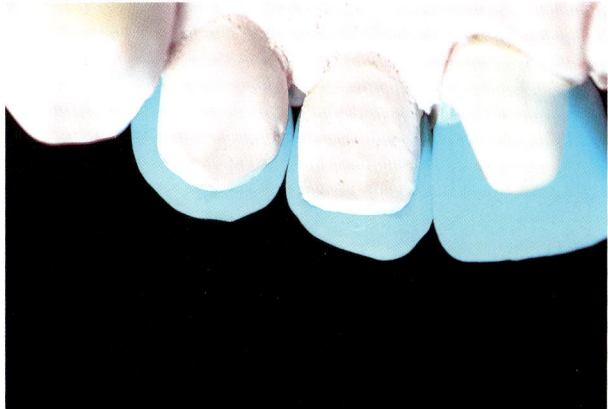

Fig 7-15 Tooth preparation, showing definitive prostheses outline: viewed from right palatal aspect.

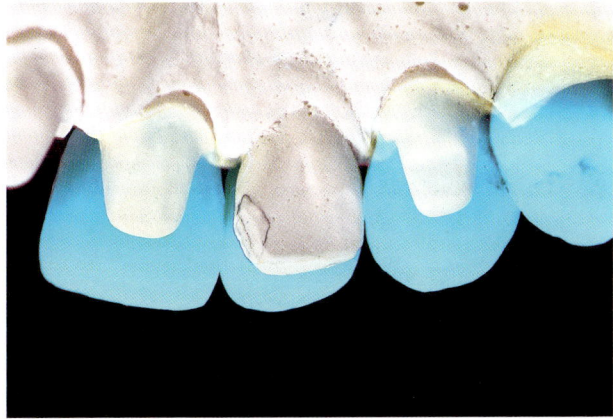

Fig 7-16 Tooth preparation, showing definitive prostheses outline: viewed from left palatal aspect.

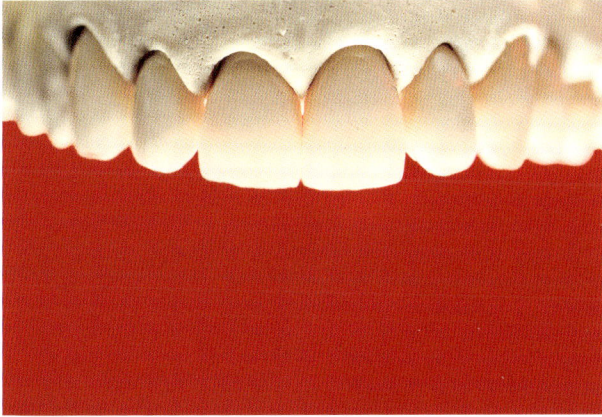

Fig 7-17 Completed definitive prostheses, showing restitution of the incisal plane curvature.

7 Restitution of Anterior Dental Esthetics with a Variety of Restorations

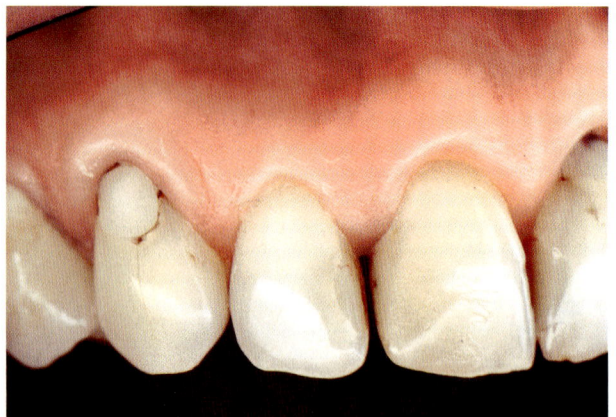

Fig 7-18 Right lateral preoperative view.

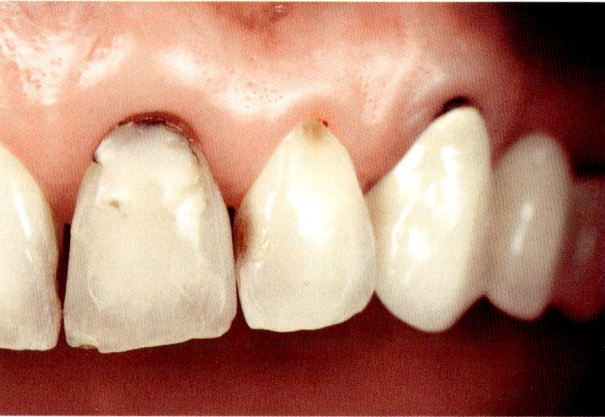

Fig 7-19 Left lateral preoperative view.

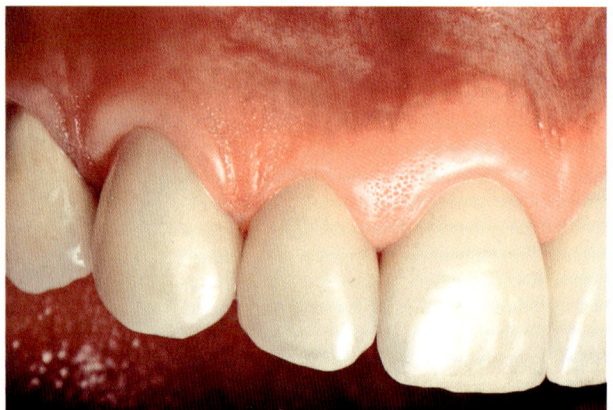

Fig 7-20 Right lateral postoperative view.

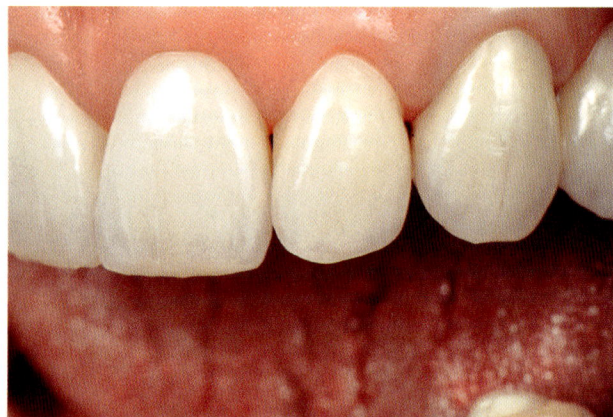

Fig 7-21 Left lateral postoperative view.

- Periodontal health has been improved – demonstrated by the stippling of the attached gingivae, the gingival groove, the healthy pink shade, and the knife-edge free gingival margin surrounding the restorations.
- The three different types of restoration (PLVs, full-coverage all-ceramic crowns, and metal-ceramic FPD) have integrated impeccably.
- The incisal plane is parallel with the curvature of the lower lip.
- The PLVs on the mandibular central incisors have restored the mandibular incisal plane.
- The free gingival margin around the maxillary right central incisor is more coronal than that around the left central incisor. However, the lip line conceals this aberration during a relaxed smile, thereby obviating the need for periodontal surgical correction.

7 Restitution of Anterior Dental Esthetics with a Variety of Restorations

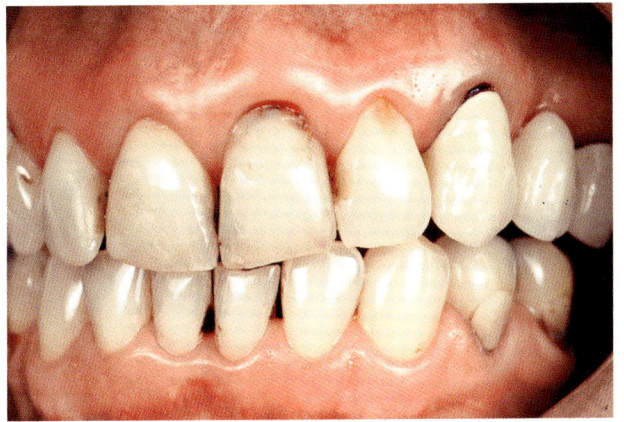
Fig 7-22 Preoperative anterior view.

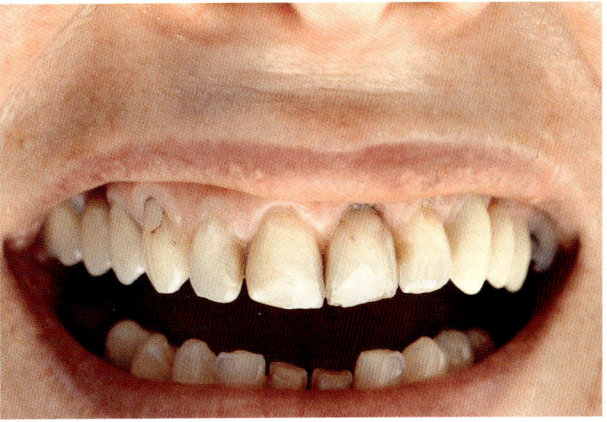
Fig 7-23 Preoperative dento-facial view.

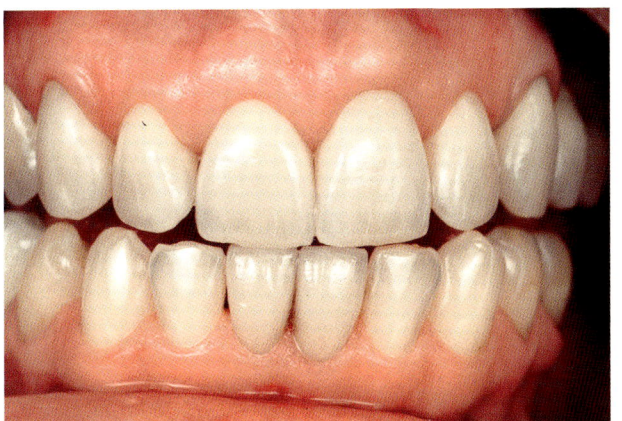
Fig 7-24 Postoperative anterior view.

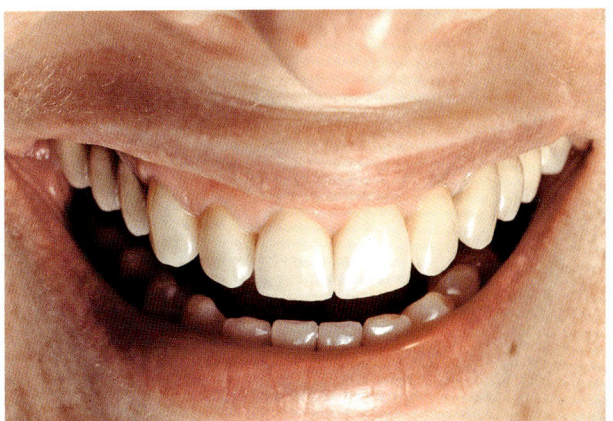
Fig 7-25 Postoperative dento-facial view.

- The maxillary dental midline is slightly misaligned, which mitigates a monotonous porcelain corridor. Introducing slight imperfections adds interest to a dental composition and detracts from a sense of artificiality.
- The facial images demonstrate not only a rejuvenated smile but also a revitalized persona.

7 Restitution of Anterior Dental Esthetics with a Variety of Restorations

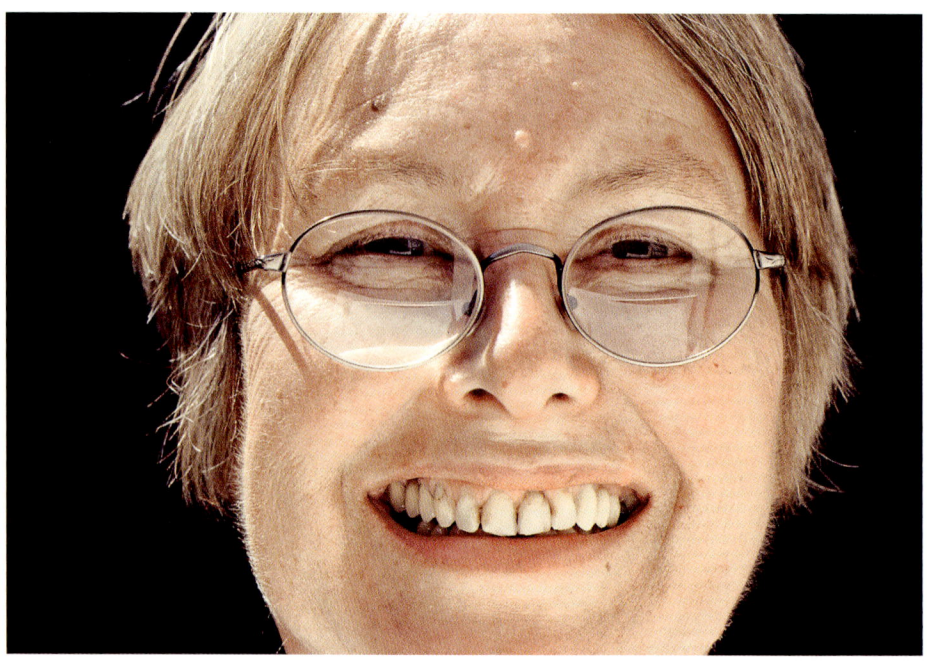

Fig 7-26 Preoperative facial view.

Discussion

The final result achieves the HFA triad objectives:
- Health – periodontium and tooth integrity.
- Function – phonetics and occlusion.
- Aesthetics – restitution of incisal plane, improved tooth morphology, elimination of black triangles, and harmonious integration of different types of restoration and restorative material.

7 Restitution of Anterior Dental Esthetics with a Variety of Restorations

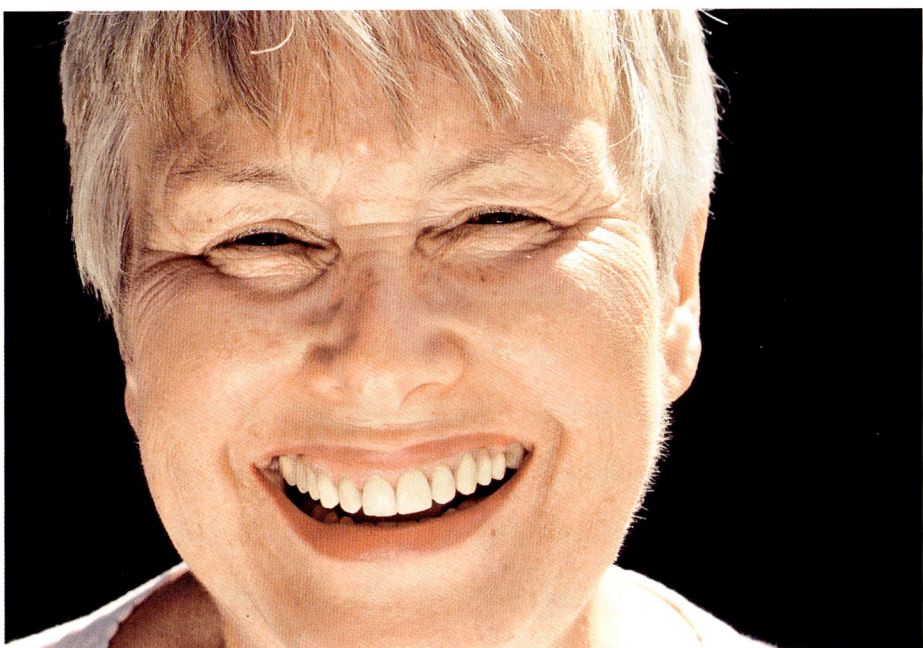

Fig 7-27 Postoperative facial view.

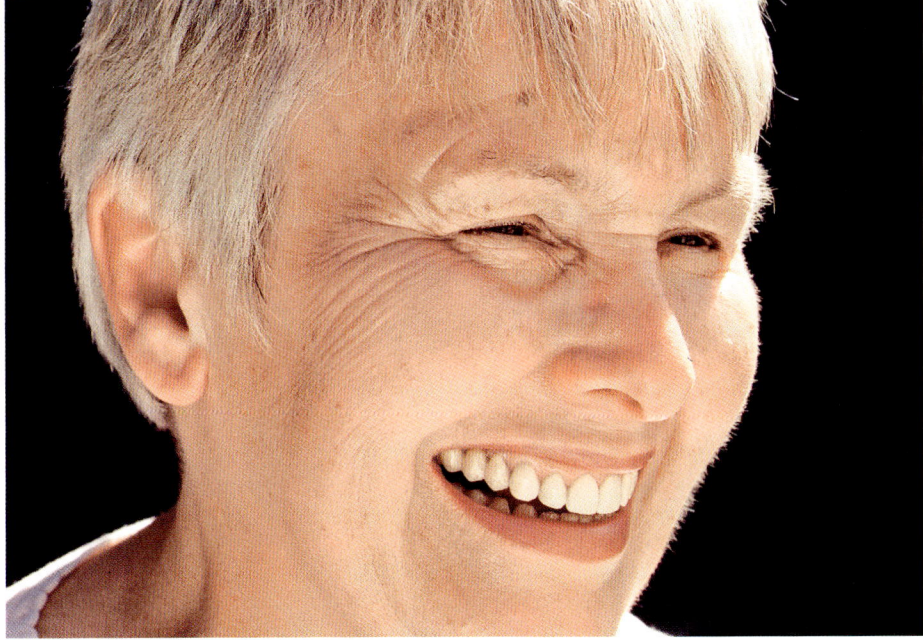

Fig 7-28 Postoperative facial view.

A Single Maxillary Central Incisor with a Hopeless Prognosis

Ceramics by Gérald Ubassy, Avignon, France

Pre- and Postoperative Status

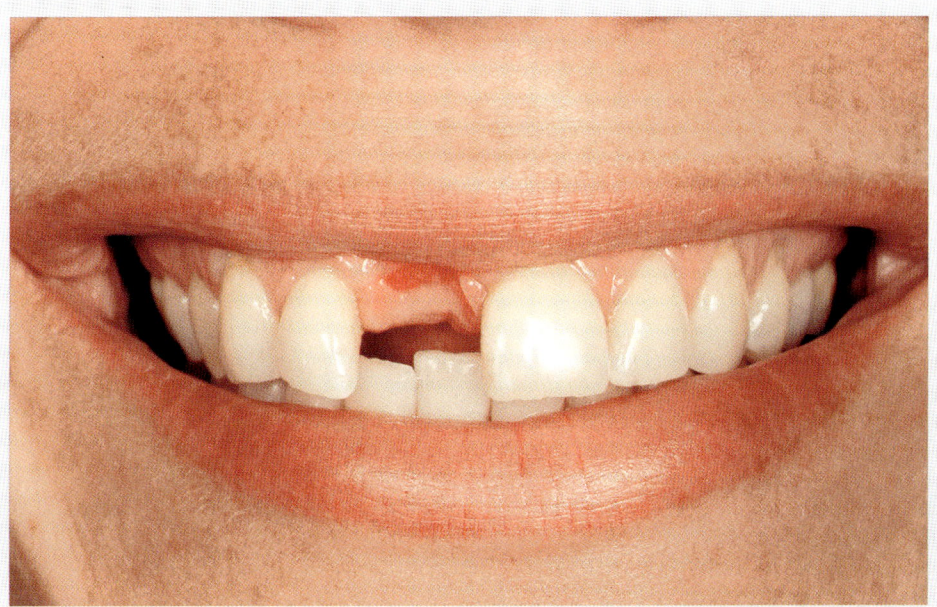

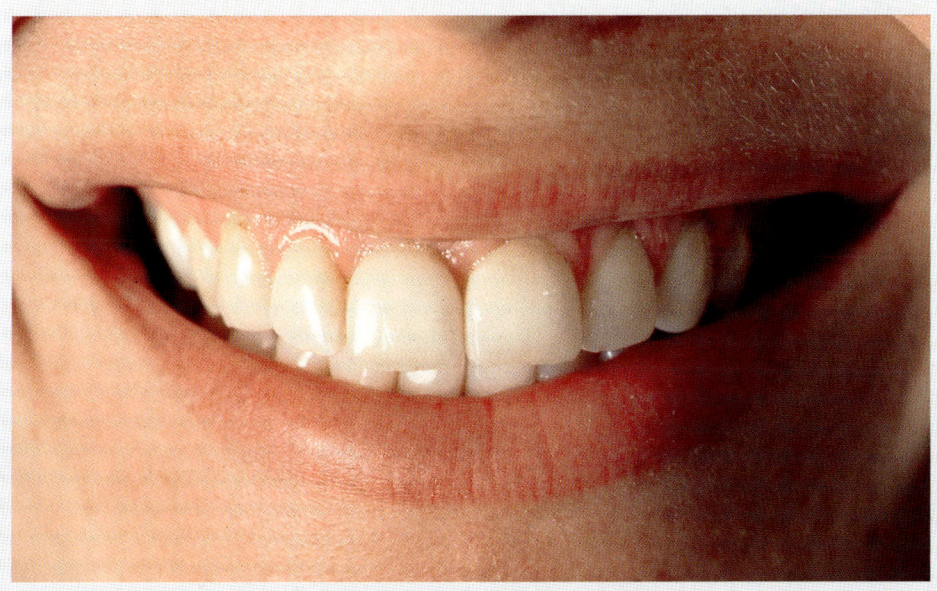

8 A Single Maxillary Central Incisor with a Hopeless Prognosis

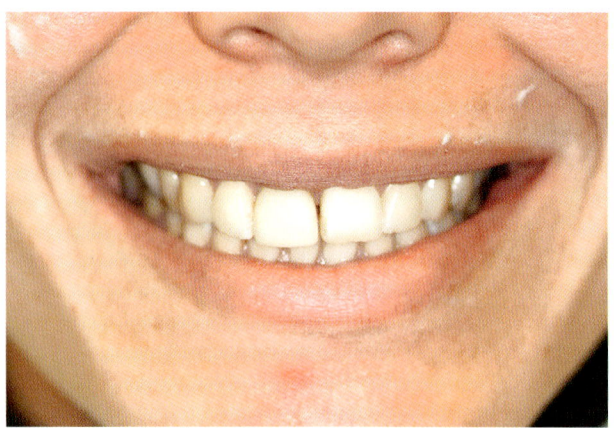

Fig 8-1 Dento-facial view of the initial metal-ceramic crown on the maxillary right central incisor and the median maxillary diastema.

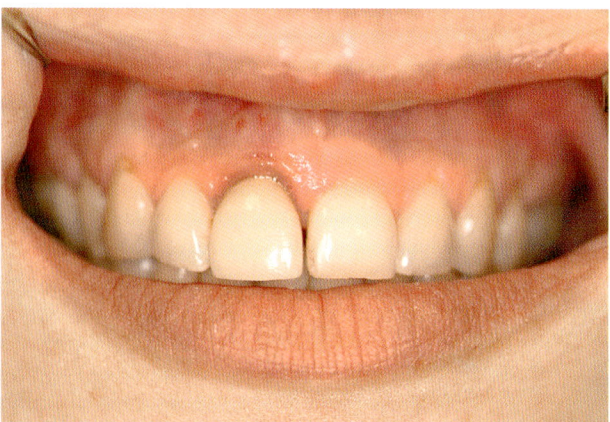

Fig 8-2 Frontal view the initial metal-ceramic crown on the maxillary right central incisor and the median maxillary diastema.

Dental History

The patient, a 29-year-old woman, attended the practice in 2005 with a missing maxillary right central incisor. She was wearing a removable acrylic-resin single-tooth partial denture. The dental history revealed that a metal-ceramic crown had been provided for the right central incisor, following repeated replacement of defective composite fillings (Figs 8-1 and 8-2). The crown was unsightly, with cervical gingival shadowing and a median maxillary diastema. A periapical radiograph shows grossly defective open crown margins, which led to inevitable endodontic complications (Fig 8-3). Subsequently, the tooth was beleaguered with consecutive failed root treatments and sporadic episodes of acute and chronic infection. The repeated infections resulted in erosion of the buccal alveolar plate, leaving the tooth with a hopeless prognosis.

The tooth was atraumatically extracted, ensuring that the palatal bone was undamaged. A full-thickness flap revealed loss of the buccal bone plate (Figs 8-4 and 8-5). This loss caused gingival recession on the buccal aspect, compromising esthetics and future reparative therapy (Figs 8-6 to 8-10). After suturing, an interim acrylic-resin removable partial denture was provided, pending further treatment (Fig 8-11).

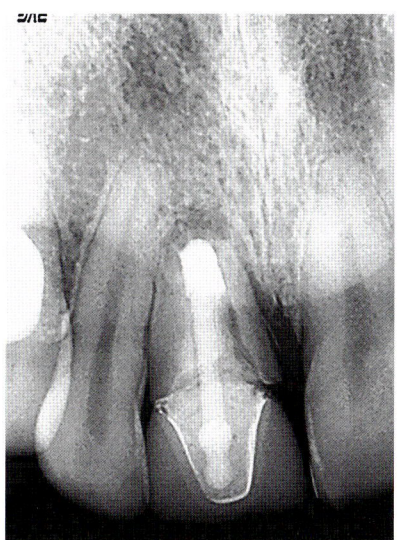

Fig 8-3 Radiograph showing the root-filled right central incisor with open, defective crown margins.

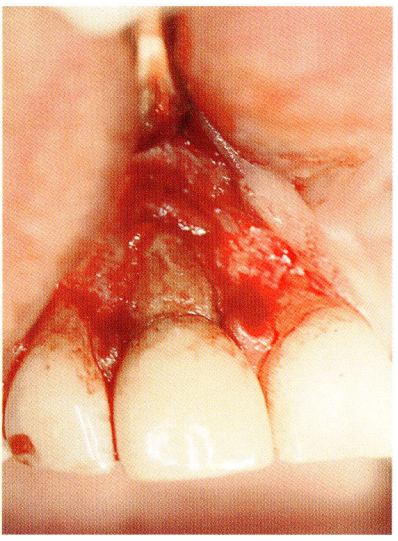

Fig 8-4 Flat elevation showing loss of buccal bone plate.

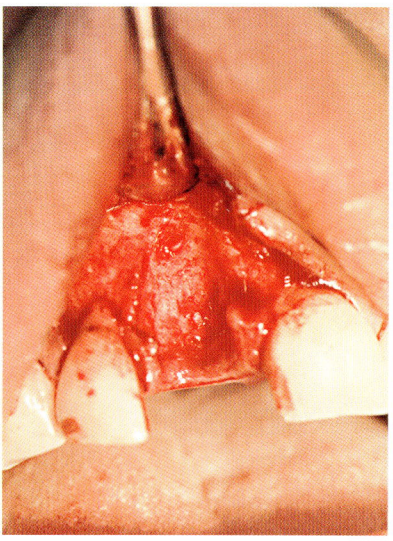

Fig 8-5 Extraction of the right central incisor.

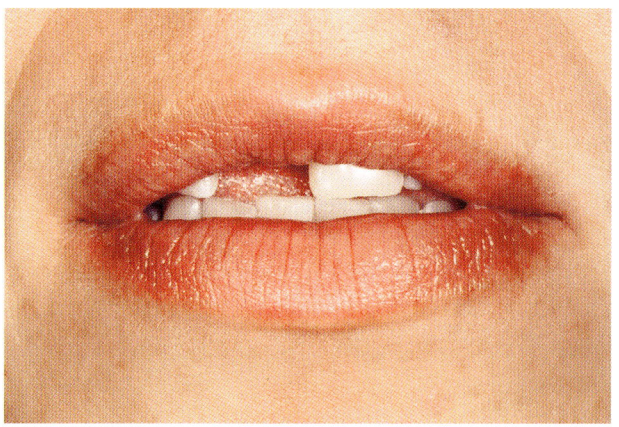

Fig 8-6 Dento-facial anterior view following extraction, at the habitual relaxed position of the lips.

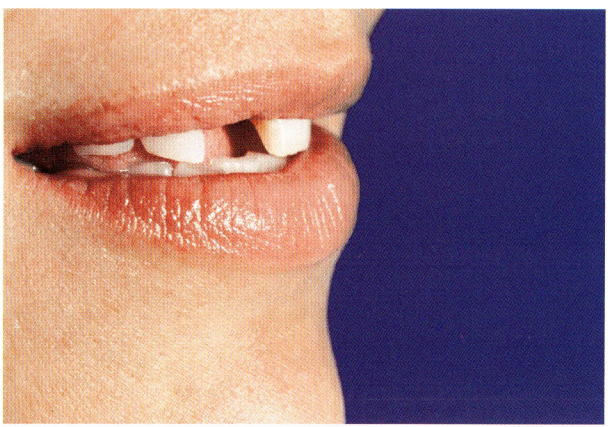

Fig 8-7 Dento-facial right lateral view following extraction, at the habitual relaxed position of the lips.

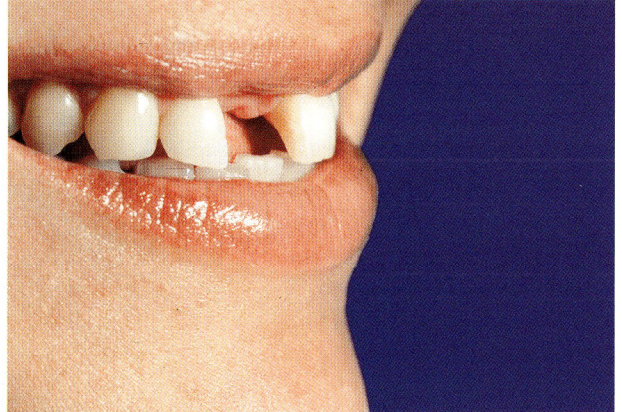

Fig 8-8 Dento-facial right lateral view following extraction, during a relaxed smile.

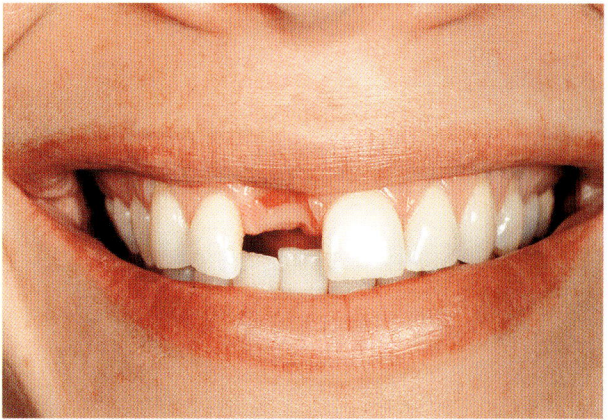

Fig 8-9 Dento-facial anterior view following extraction, during a relaxed smile.

8 A Single Maxillary Central Incisor with a Hopeless Prognosis

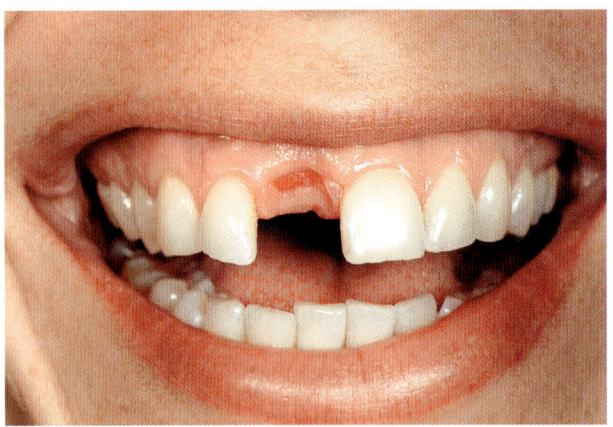

Fig 8-10 Dento-facial anterior view following extraction, during an exaggerated smile.

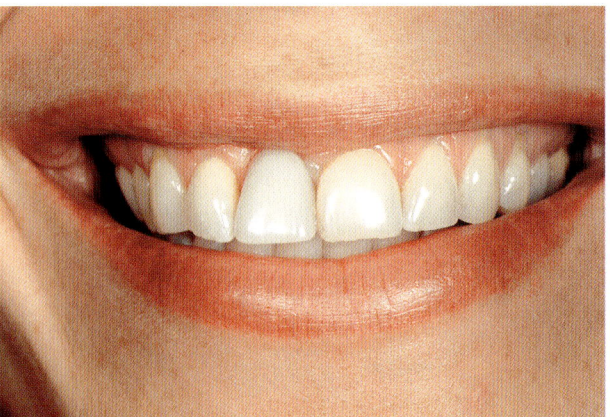

Fig 8-11 Dento-facial anterior view with the provisional acrylic-resin partial denture in situ.

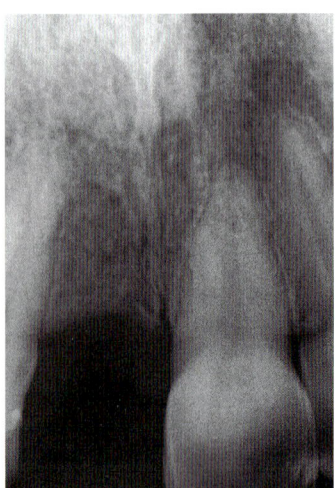

Fig 8-12 Preoperative radiograph following extraction of the right central incisor.

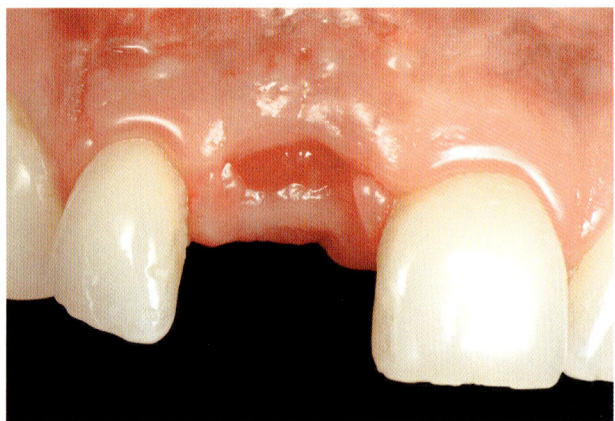

Fig 8-13 Anterior view showing recession of the buccal FGM at the extraction site.

Preoperative Status

A periapical radiograph taken at the commencement of treatment shows the healed site following extraction (Fig 8-12). The preoperative images show buccal recession of the free gingival margin (FGM) (Fig 8-13) and a steep anterior guidance (Figs 8-14 and 8-15). The mesial–distal residual space at the right central incisor site was wider than at the left central, owing to the median maxillary diastema. There was buccal collapse of the alveolar ridge, which resulted in a horizontal defect (Fig 8-16). The defect was clearly evident on the preoperative plaster cast (Fig 8-17). The lip line was high during an exaggerated smile, showing the cervical aspects of the anterior maxillary teeth (Fig 8-18).

8 A Single Maxillary Central Incisor with a Hopeless Prognosis

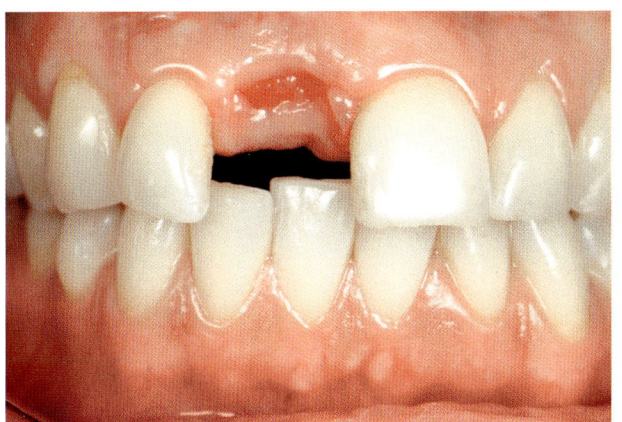

Fig 8-14 Anterior view in centric occlusion.

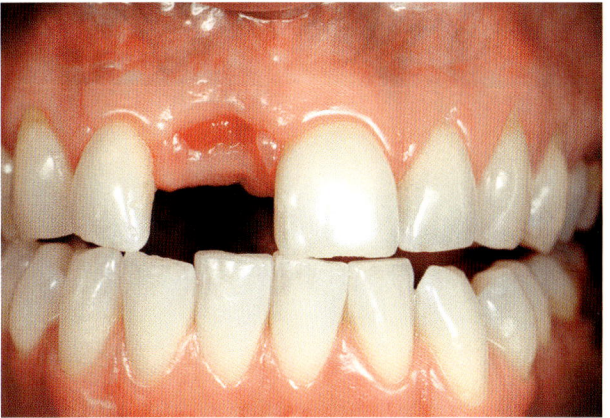

Fig 8-15 Anterior view in protrusive excursion, with a steep anterior guidance (compare with Fig 8-14).

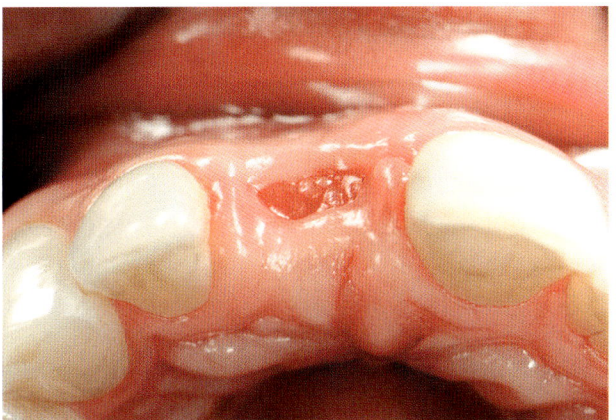

Fig 8-16 Preoperative incisal view.

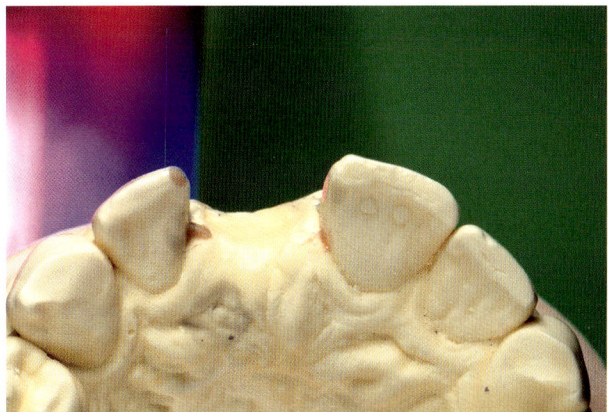

Fig 8-17 Preoperative plaster cast showing collapse of the buccal bone plate.

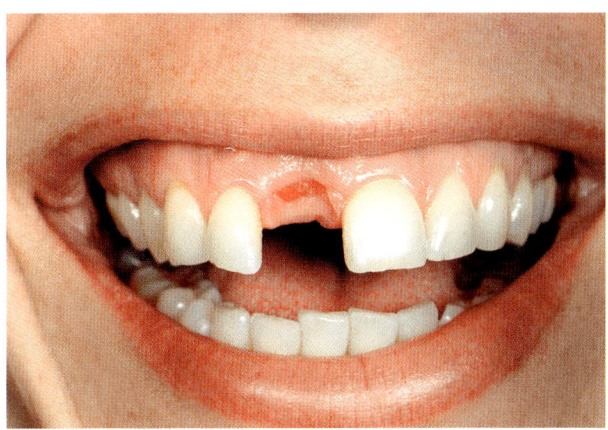

Fig 8-18 Dento-facial anterior view following extraction, during an exaggerated smile.

113

8 A Single Maxillary Central Incisor with a Hopeless Prognosis

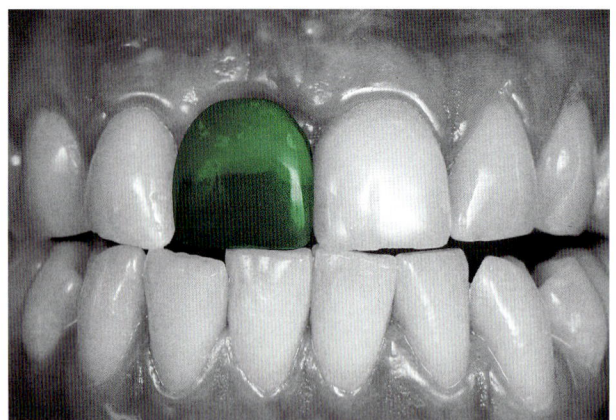

Fig 8-19 Option 1: removable acrylic-resin partial denture (green).

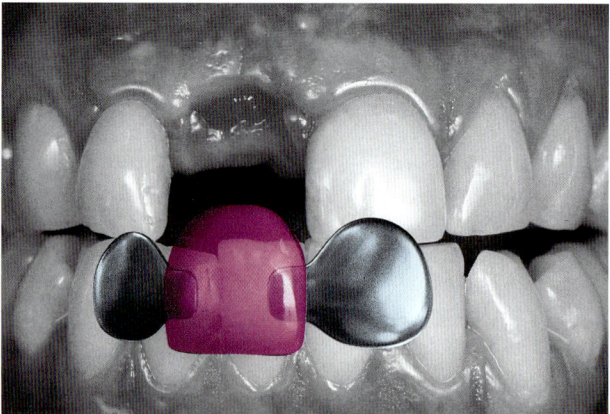

Fig 8-20 Option 2: Rochette bridge (purple) with palatal wings.

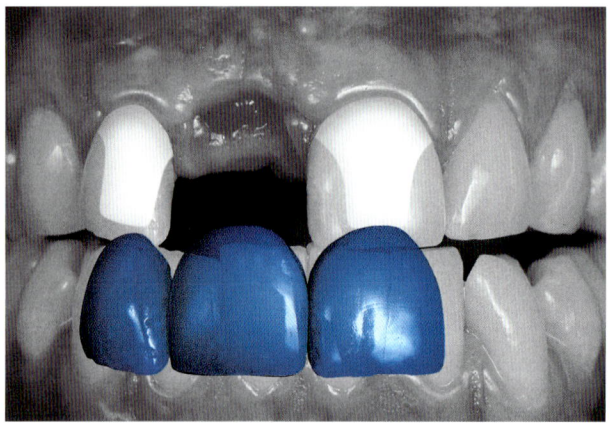

Fig 8-21 Option 3: three-unit fixed partial denture (blue), using the right lateral and left central incisors as abutments.

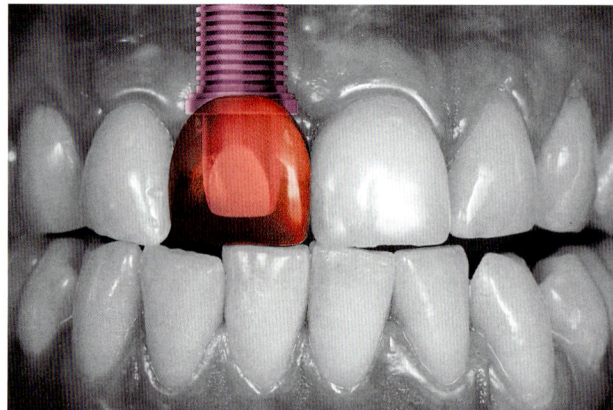

Fig 8-22 Option 4: implant-supported crown (red).

Treatment Options

1. Removable acrylic-resin partial denture (Fig 8-19).
2. Rochette bridge with palatal wings on the right lateral and left central incisors (Fig 8-20).
3. Fixed partial denture, using the right lateral and left central incisors as abutments (Fig 8-21).
4. Implant-supported crown (Fig 8-22).

Scientific Credence for Treatment Options

The removable partial denture and Rochette bridge are the least invasive options, but both would be prone to possible dislodgement. A fixed partial denture is more stable, but this would be a highly destructive option. The implant is probably the ideal fixed option, but bone and soft tissue grafting would be essential for achieving optimal esthetics. The situation is further compounded by the previous infections and reduced vascularity. Furthermore, the high lip line reveals the cervical margins of the maxillary incisors, warranting connective tissue grafting to enhance the tissue volume to compensate for gingival recession following implant fixture placement.

Clinical Erudition and Feasibility

The removable partial denture and Rochette bridge options are relatively straightforward. The implant option, however, would require some consideration. First, the buccal gingival recession combined with the collapse of the alveolar ridge mean that skill and experience would be required to rebuild both of these deficient tissues. Second, care would be needed when choosing the restorative material for the definitive crown. The crown would have to be sufficiently resilient to be capable of withstanding the steep anterior guidance.

Patient Needs and Wants

The patient refused the removable denture option. She disliked her interim acrylic-resin prosthesis and felt that a removable denture would be socially embarrassing. The Rochette bridge was rejected on the grounds of instability, while a fixed partial denture was considered too destructive. In addition, the patient had initially lost the right central incisor through a defective crown and so did not wish to have other healthy teeth filed down, which could also result in endodontic compromises or extractions.

The implant option was the most appealing to the patient. She understood that treatment would be protracted, and that she may have to accept a soft tissue esthetic compromise if connective tissue grafting did not achieve ideal "pink esthetics" around the implant-supported crown.

Treatment Sequence

The first point that the patient wished to address was the median maxillary diastema. The diastema was congenital, as shown by the photographs of the patient when she was 8 years of age (Fig 8-23), in her teens (Fig 8-24), early twenties (Fig 8-25), and late twenties (Fig 8-26). Furthermore, the initial crown on the right central incisor maintained this space (see Figs 8-1 and 8-2). However, as she was having a new crown, she now wished to close the diastema. As mentioned above, the residual space at the right central incisor site was

8 A Single Maxillary Central Incisor with a Hopeless Prognosis

Fig 8-23 Patient at 8 years of age. Notice the median maxillary diastema.

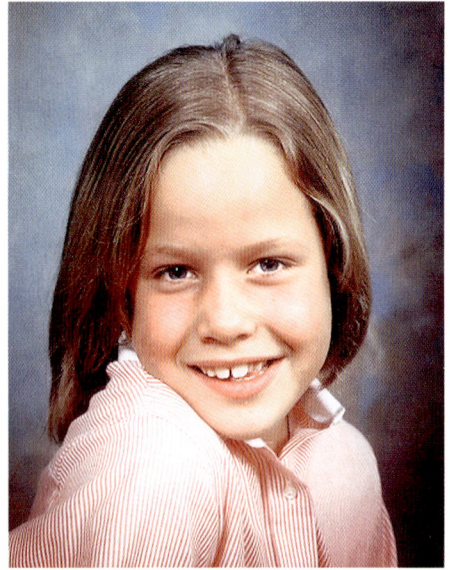
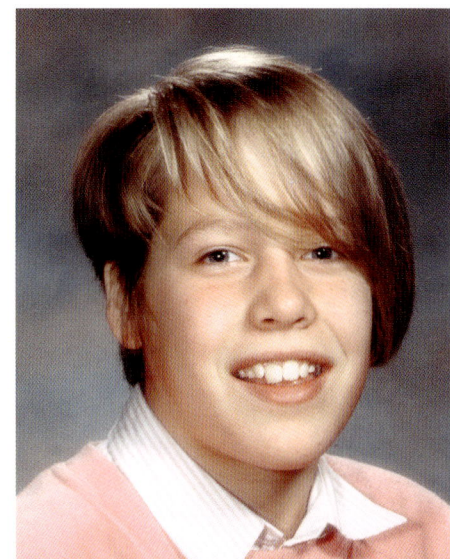

Fig 8-24 Patient in her teens.

Fig 8-25 Patient in her early twenties.

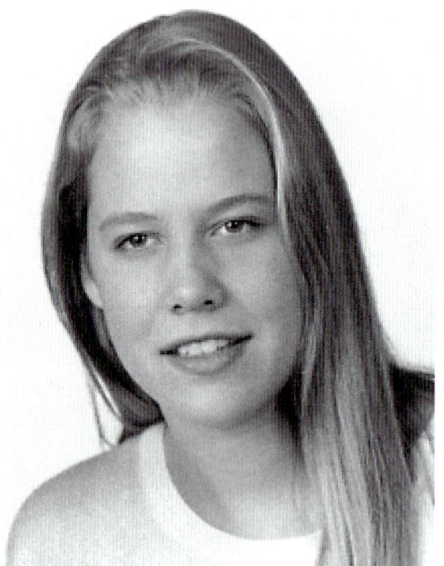
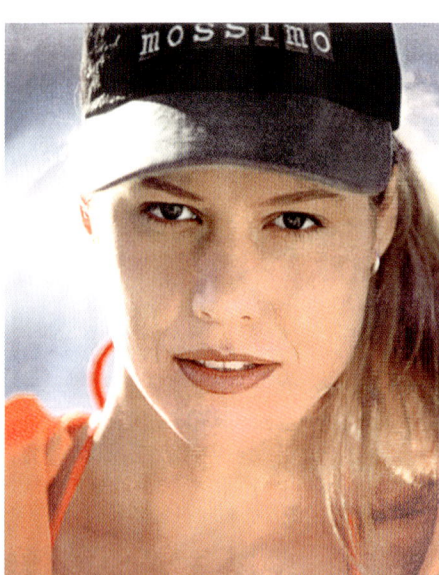

Fig 8-26 Patient in her late twenties.

slightly larger than at the left central, and so would result in a wider tooth. Nevertheless, the patient was willing to accept this concession. A shade analysis was performed, using three different shade guides, to ascertain and match the shade of the new crown to the surrounding teeth (Figs 8-27 to 8-29).

In September 2005, the implant fixture (RP Nobel Replace) was placed concurrently with bone grafting using Bio-Oss. A few months later, soft tissue grafting was carried out using connective tissue from the palate to bulk out the alveolar ridge on the buccal aspect (Fig 8-30). Pre- and postgrafting plaster casts demonstrate the coronal gain in vertical soft tissue height of the FGM at the right central incisor site (Figs 8-31 and 8-32).

8 A Single Maxillary Central Incisor with a Hopeless Prognosis

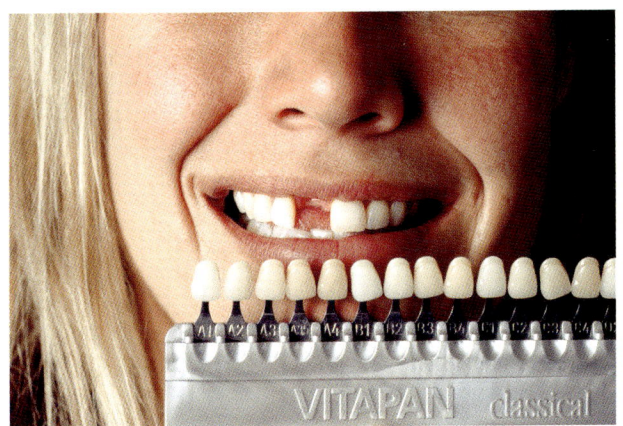

Fig 8-27 Shade analysis using the Vita Classical shade guide.

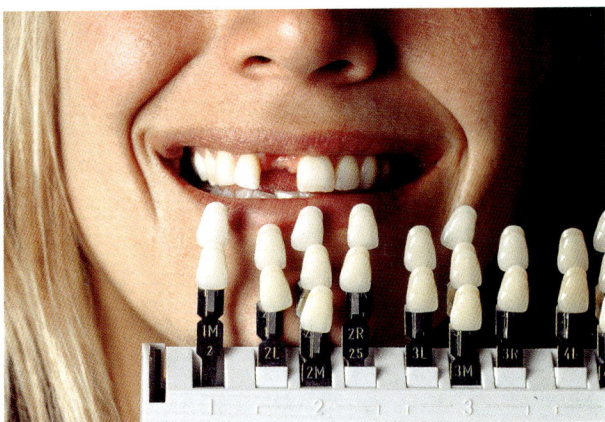

Fig 8-28 Shade analysis using the Vita 3D shade guide.

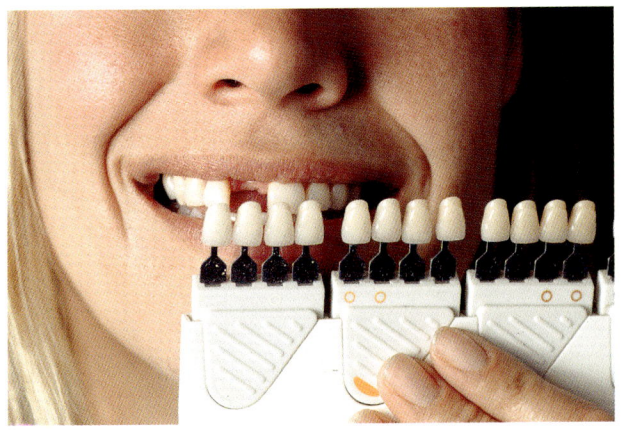

Fig 8-29 Shade analysis using the Ivolcar-Vivadent Chromascop shade guide.

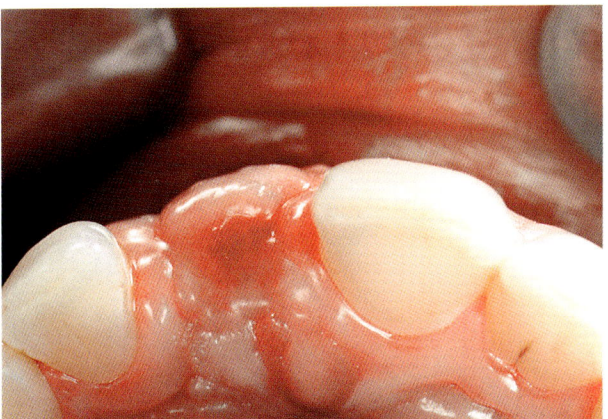

Fig 8-30 Incisal view showing connective tissue augmentation of the right central incisor site.

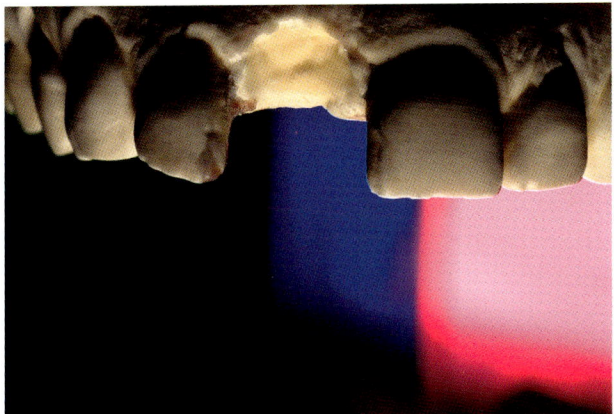

Fig 8-31 Preoperative plaster cast with apical position of the FGM at the right central incisor site.

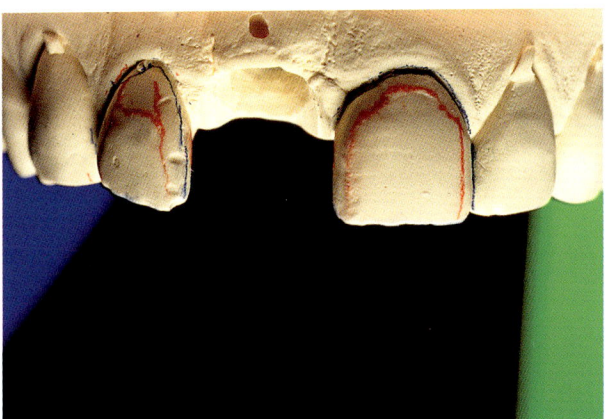

Fig 8-32 Plaster cast with coronal position of the FGM at the right central incisor site following connective tissue grafting.

117

8 A Single Maxillary Central Incisor with a Hopeless Prognosis

Fig 8-33 Preoperative radiograph: September 2005.

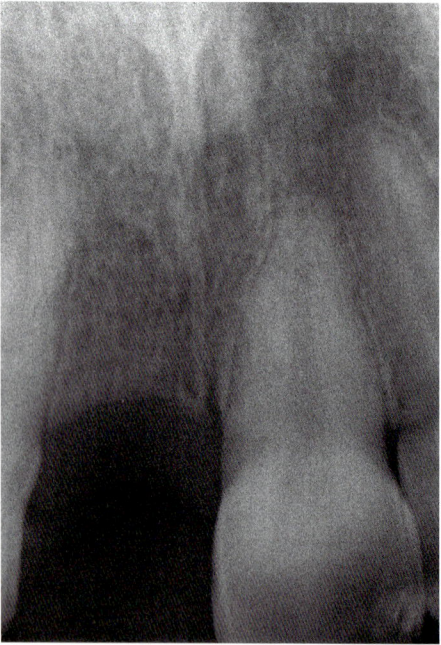

Fig 8-34 Radiograph following implant fixture placement, with the titanium abutment and the provisional crown at the right central incisor site: April 2006.

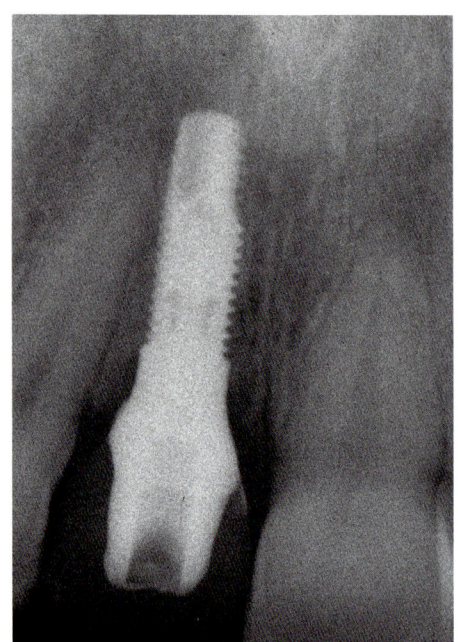

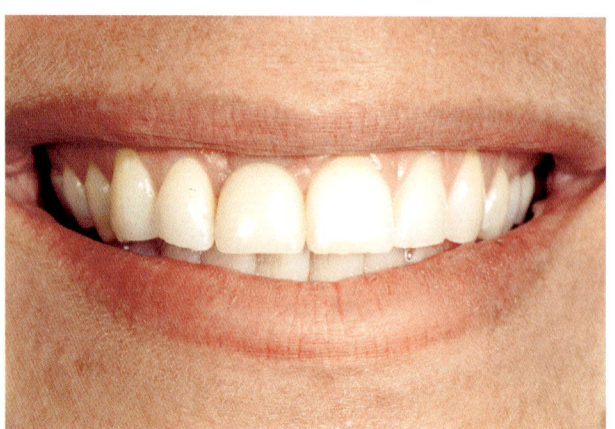

Fig 8-35 Dento-facial view with the provisional crown in situ at the right central incisor site.

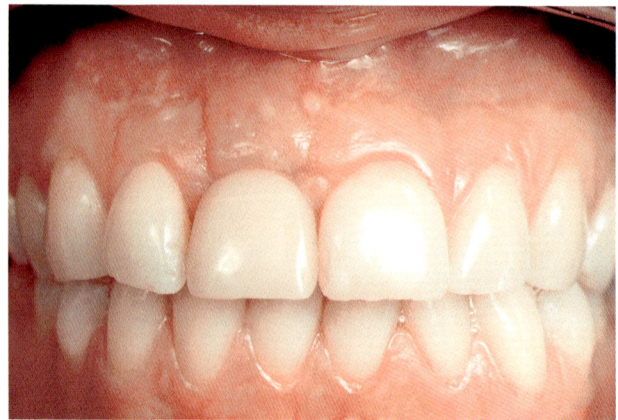

Fig 8-36 Anterior view with the provisional crown in situ at the right central incisor site: centric occlusion.

Radiographs from September 2005 and April 2006 are shown in Figure 8-33 and Figure 8-34, respectively. The removable partial denture, which the patient loathed, was discarded and replaced with a resin-composite provisional crown supported by a titanium abutment. The crown was worn for 6 months and periodically adjusted to finalize the form and occlusion and to sculpt the connective tissue graft (Figs 8-35 to 8-40).

In October 2006, impressions were made for the definitive zirconia abutment and crown (Figs 8-41 to 8-44). An Empress 2 (Ivolcar-Vivadent, Liechtenstein) was chosen for improved light transmission to avoid cervical shadowing, which was also mitigated by using a custom zirconia abutment (Figs 8-45 to 8-47).

8 A Single Maxillary Central Incisor with a Hopeless Prognosis

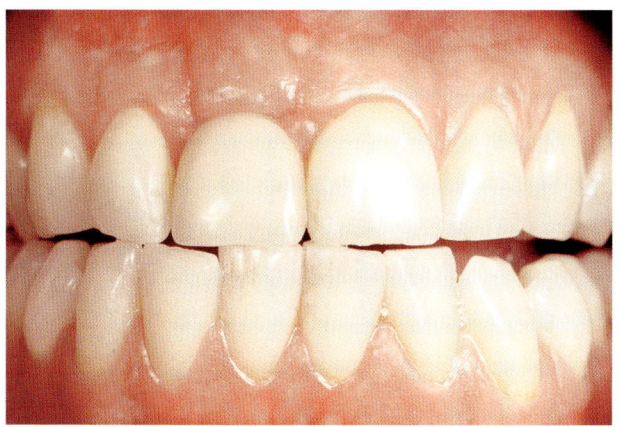

Fig 8-37 Anterior view with the provisional crown in situ at the right central incisor site: protrusion.

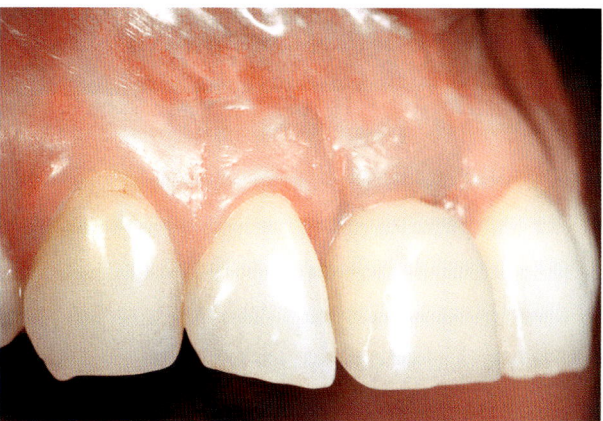

Fig 8-38 Right lateral view of the provisional crown in situ at the right central incisor site.

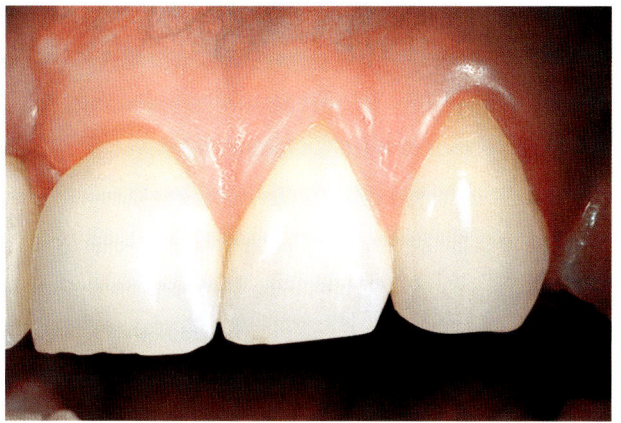

Fig 8-39 Left lateral view: compare the facial soft tissue bulk around natural left central incisor with that around the provisional crown on the right central incisor site (Fig 8-38).

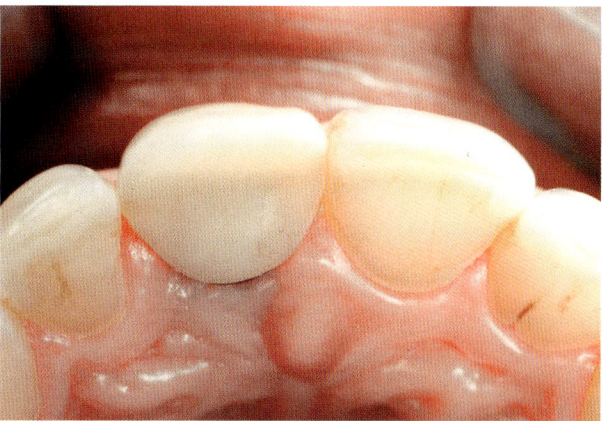

Fig 8-40 Incisal view of the provisional crown in situ at the right central incisor site.

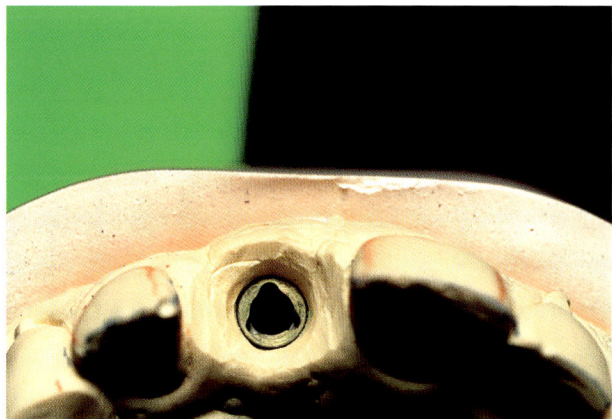

Fig 8-41 Plaster cast with the implant analogue at the right central incisor site: incisal view.

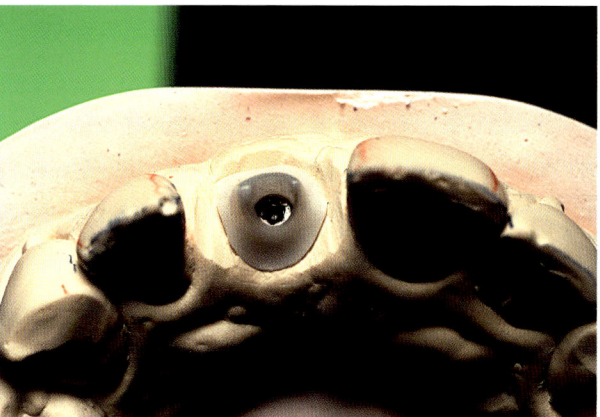

Fig 8-42 Plaster cast with the zirconia abutment: incisal view.

8 A Single Maxillary Central Incisor with a Hopeless Prognosis

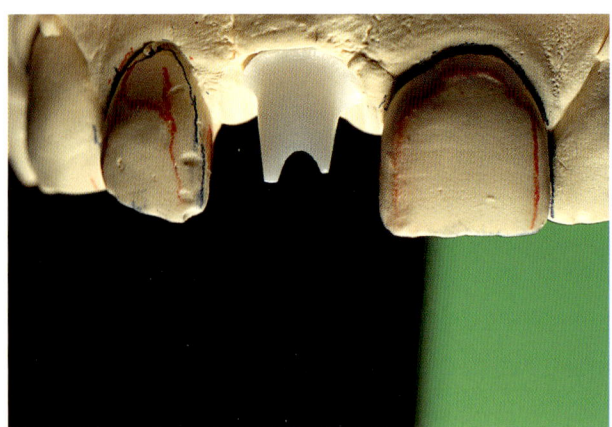

Fig 8-43 Plaster cast with the zirconia abutment: anterior view.

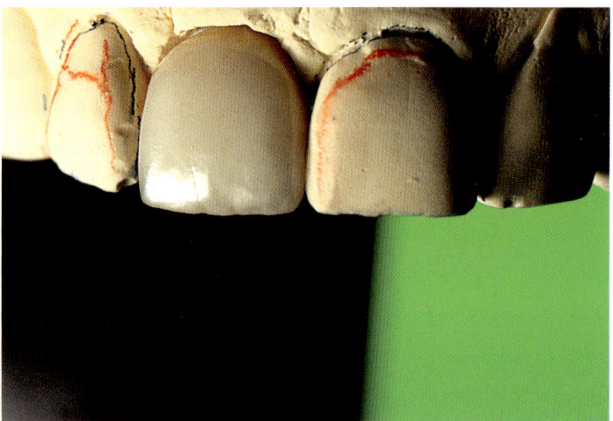

Fig 8-44 Plaster cast with the definitive crown: anterior view.

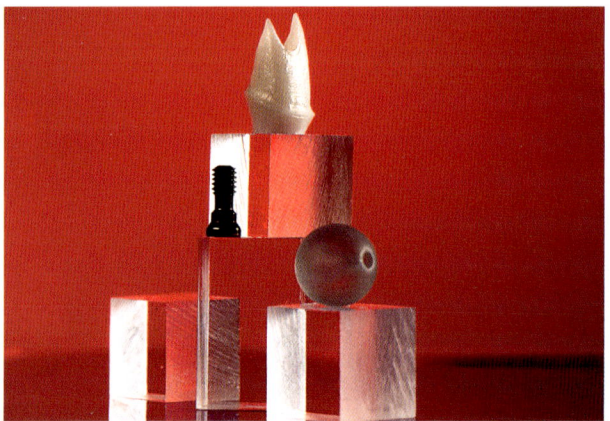

Fig 8-45 Zirconia abutment and fixing screw.

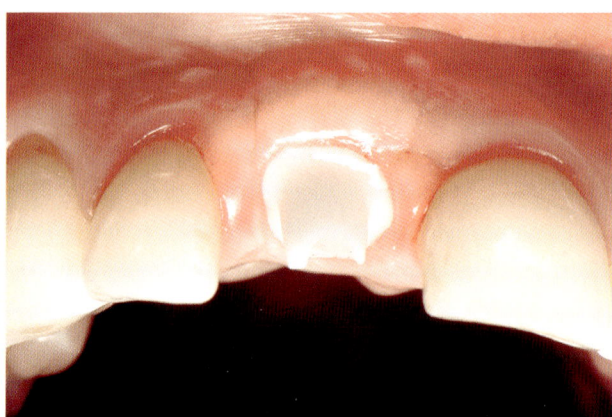

Fig 8-46 Zirconia abutment screwed on to the implant fixture: inciso-anterior view.

Upon delivery, the crown was cemented; the postoperative views are shown in Figures 8-48 to 8-52. A detailed analysis (Figs 8-53 and 8-54) shows:
- closure of the maxillary median diastema, with acceptable mesial–distal proportions of the crown
- presence of the maxillary median interproximal papilla
- acceptable color match of crown with adjacent teeth.

The pre- and postoperative dento-facial and facial views are shown in Figures 8-55 to 8-58. The superb crown esthetics are attributed to the meticulously incorporation of characterizations and incisal-edge undulations, similar to the natural left central incisor. Viewed from a social distance, the smile is radiant, and it is difficult to isolate the artificial crown from the neighboring natural dentition.

8 A Single Maxillary Central Incisor with a Hopeless Prognosis

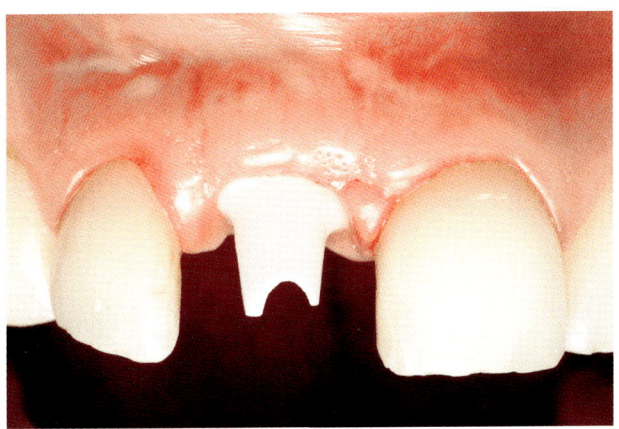

Fig 8-47 Zirconia abutment screwed onto the implant fixture: anterior view.

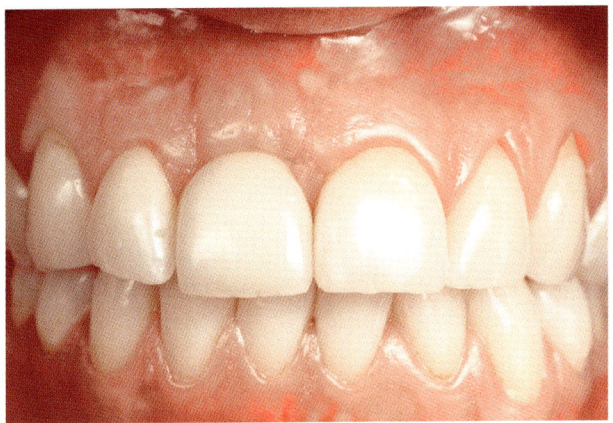

Fig 8-48 Implant-supported cement-retained definitive crown at the right central incisor site: centric occlusion. Notice the closure of the median maxillary diastema.

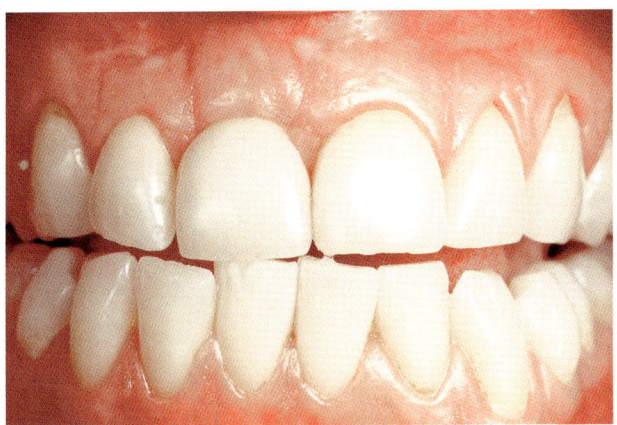

Fig 8-49 Implant-supported cement-retained definitive crown at right central incisor site: protrusive. Notice closure of median maxillary diastema.

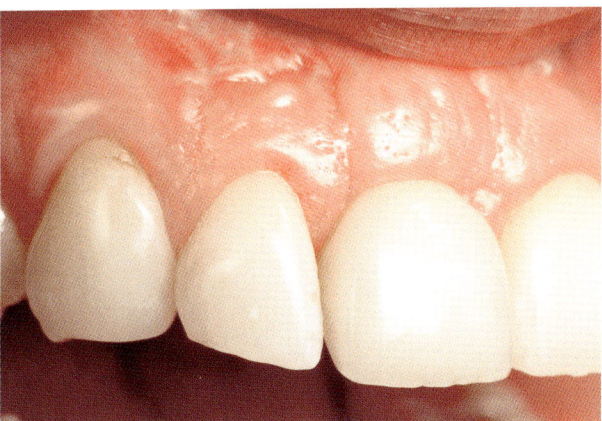

Fig 8-50 Right lateral view showing the maturing connective tissue graft at the right central incisor site.

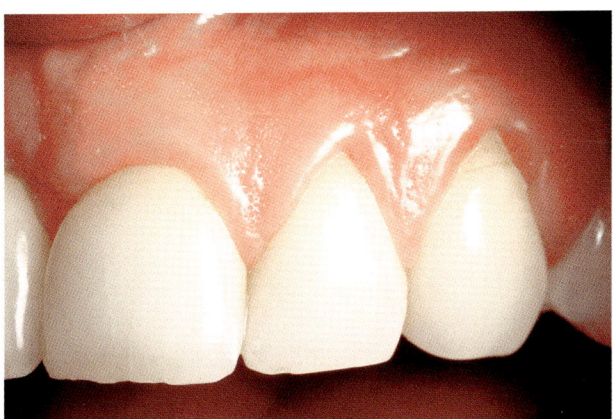

Fig 8-51 Left lateral view: compare the soft tissue bulk around the natural left central incisor with the contralateral site (Fig 8-50).

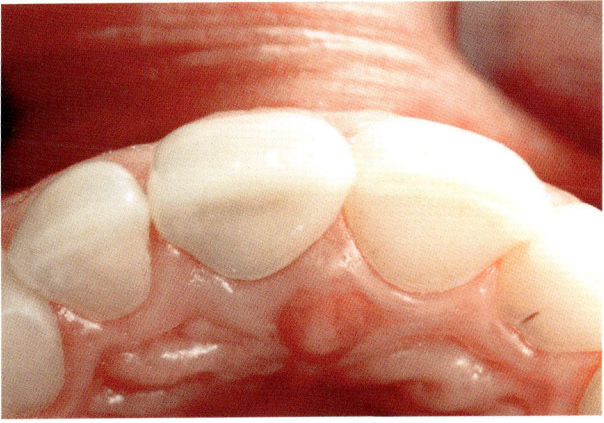

Fig 8-52 Implant-supported cement-retained definitive crown at the right central incisor site: incisal view.

8 A Single Maxillary Central Incisor with a Hopeless Prognosis

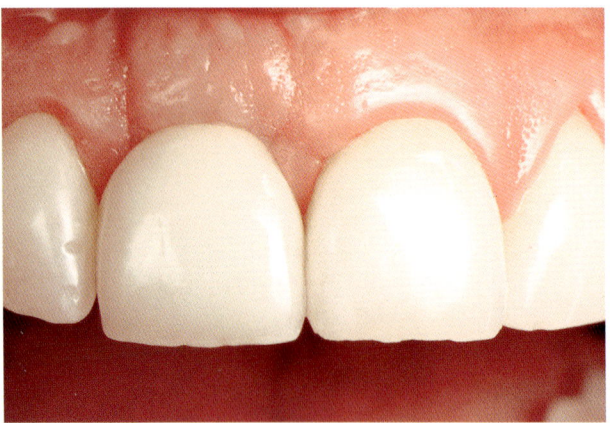

Fig 8-53 Implant-supported cement-retained definitive crown at the right central incisor site: anterior view.

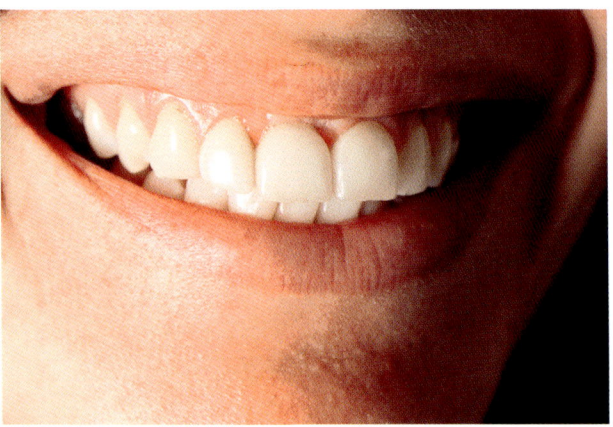

Fig 8-54 Implant-supported cement-retained definitive crown at the right central incisor site: dento-facial view.

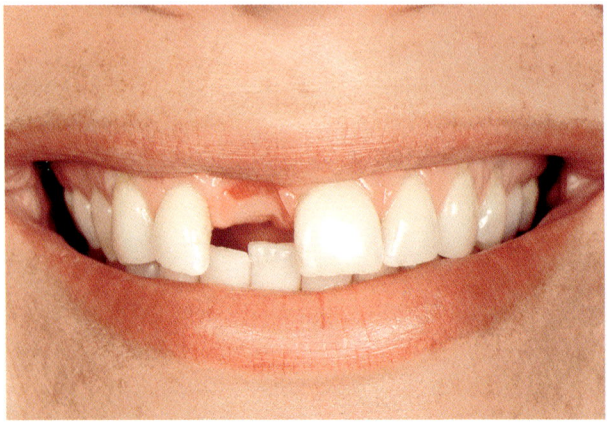

Fig 8-55 Preoperative dento-facial view during a relaxed smile.

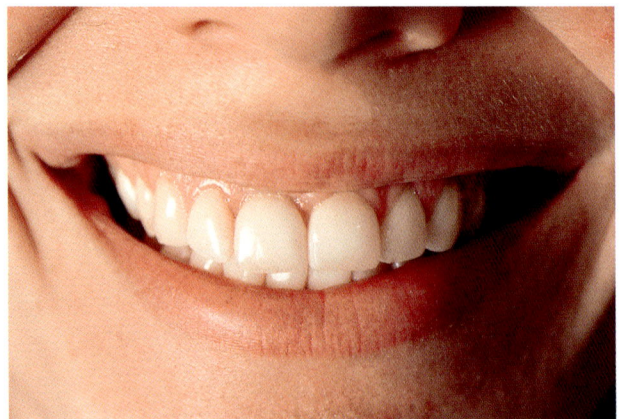

Fig 8-56 Postoperative dento-facial view during a relaxed smile.

Discussion

Most of the problems with this case study stemmed from the buccal bone plate erosion, caused by the repeated chronic infections associated with the maxillary right central incisor. The bone and soft tissues grafts might have been superfluous had the buccal plate been present. If the buccal plate is intact, it is paramount to extract failing or fractured teeth with minimal trauma, and efforts should be made to retain the alveolar housing and to minimize trauma to the soft tissues.

8 A Single Maxillary Central Incisor with a Hopeless Prognosis

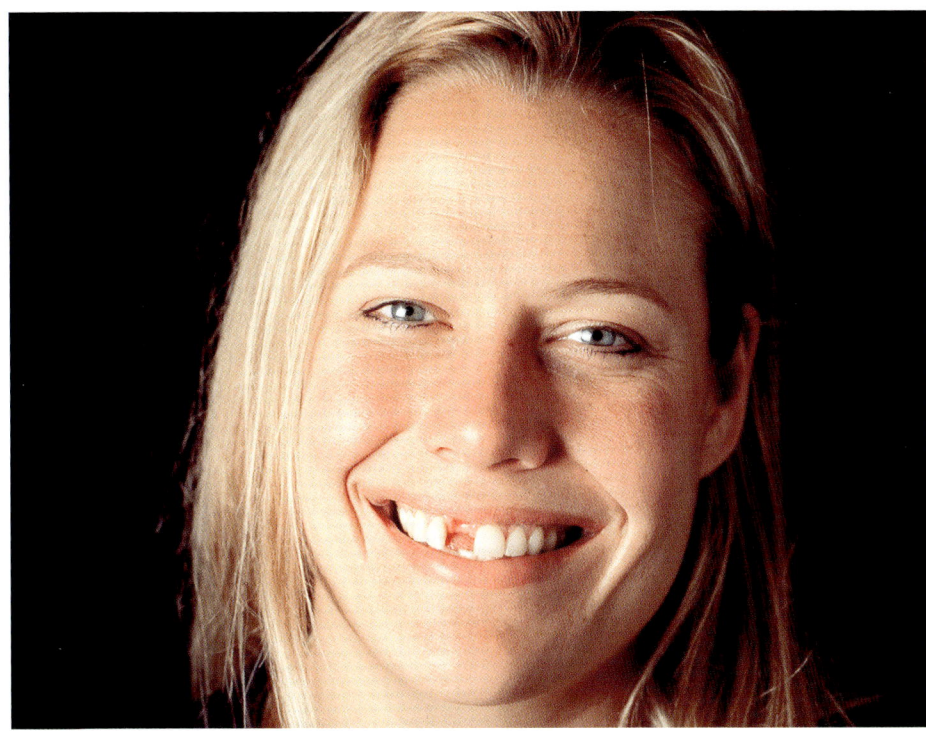

Fig 8-57 Preoperative facial view.

Fig 8-58 Postoperative facial view.

A repeatedly infected site usually has reduced vascularity, and implant placement should be delayed until bone grafting has integrated and new blood vessels have colonized the exsanguinated site. Hence, this patient was not a suitable candidate for immediate implant placement at the time of extraction. The bone grafting was concurrent with implant placement because the tooth had been extracted some months earlier, allowing the site to heal. It was, therefore, anticipated that the time lapse between extraction and the implant placement would have allowed vascularization.

The postoperative result shows scarring at the site of the connective tissue graft. Scarring is more prevalent when the dental biotype is thick (as in this woman), predisposing to scarring owing to an abundance of fibrous tissue. Another point worth noting is that the gingival zenith around the crown is more coronal than that around the natural left central incisor. Had the patient been fastidious, this could have been rectified, together with the scarring, by using a soft tissue laser.

Occlusion was a crucial factor in this case study, and it is worth mentioning that the provisional crown dislodged on several occasions and had to be adjusted and recemented. For this reason, the choice of material for the definitive crown is debatable. Owing to the steep anterior guidance, a metal-ceramic crown would be an ideal choice, but it would yield poor esthetics. Therefore, strength was compromised for esthetics by using an all-ceramic system. Empress 2, with a flexural strength of approximately 350 MPa, is stronger than conventional silica-based ceramics, but it is not the strongest ceramic on the market. A stronger ceramic, such as alumina or zirconia, may have been a better choice, with flexural strengths of 700 MPa and 1,000 MPa, respectively.

Index

A

abrasion 22
aesthetics *see* esthetics
alumina ceramics 60, 124
anterior Dahl appliance 37
anterior deprogrammer 37
apicectomies 65–67, 68, 93
    advantages 72
    disadvantages 72, 93
attrition 22
autonomy 5

B

beneficence 5
bio-col technique 74
"black triangles" 87, 96
bleaching 82–83, 96–97
buccal bone plate loss 110–111, 122
buccal reduction 26, 29

C

cantilever bridges
    advantages 12, 72
    disadvantages 12, 44, 72
    prior to implant 45, 47
ceramic prostheses 60, 124
cervical margins, for PLVs 31
cervical shadowing 14, 102, 118
CLVs *see* composite laminate veneers
communication breakdown 90
composite fillings
    disadvantages 96
    replacement 96–97, 110
composite laminate veneers (CLVs) 22
    advantages 25
    disadvantages 25
    PLVs vs 25
cost of treatment 7
creep 48
crowns
    deficient margin rectification 87
    definitive 44, 49, 82–84, 115, 118–124
    full-coverage 22, 100, 104
    provisional 48–49, 77–83, 118–119, 124

D

declining maxillary incisors 39–54
    clinical erudition and feasibility 44
    dental history 40
    discussion 51–53
    patient needs and wants 44–45
    postoperative status 39, 51–54
    preoperative status 39–42, 51–54
    scientific credence for treatment 44
    treatment options 42–43
    treatment sequence 45–51
dentin sealing 91
dietary advice 25
discoloration, progressive 68–71
duration of treatment 7

E

Empress 2 crowns 84, 118, 124
erosion 22
esthetics 4, 96, 106
ethics 5
evidence-based (EB) treatment planning 1–8
    clinical erudition and feasibility 5–7
    factors 2–3
    scientific rationale 3–5
    as triangle 2–3
experience 6

F

feather-edge reduction 28–29, 30
fibrin 20
fixed partial dentures (FPDs)
    advantages 12, 58, 115
    disadvantages 12, 44, 58, 72, 115
    materials 60, 100
    treatment sequences using 60–61, 99–105
    see also traumatic loss of maxillary central incisors
function 4, 96, 106

H

healing caps 77–78
health 3, 96, 106
HFA triad 4, 96, 106
hydrofluoric acid 34

Index

I

implant abutments
    materials 16, 20
    shape 16–17
    see also titanium abutments; zirconia abutments
implants
    advantages 12, 72, 115
    disadvantages 12, 44, 72, 115
    treatment sequences using 13–19, 45–51, 74–91, 115–122
    see also declining maxillary incisors
incisal edge reduction 28–29, 30, 31
intaglio surface pretreatment 33–34
interproximal contacts 31–35
IPS e.max crowns 89–90

J

justice 5

K

knowledge 5

L

Le Forte fracture, planned 58, 59
locking taper implant design 20
lower arch realignment
    advantages 44
    disadvantages 44
luting agents 32

M

maxilliary central incisors *see* restitution of anterior dental esthetics
maxillary canines
    simulating as lateral incisors 71, 87
    see also replacing maxillary canines and lateral incisors; restitution of anterior dental esthetics
maxillary central incisors
    extraction 74–76, 110–112
    see also declining maxillary incisors; restitution of anterior dental esthetics; single maxillary central incisor with hopeless prognosis; traumatic loss of maxillary central incisors; vicissitudes of maxillary incisors
maxillary lateral incisors *see* declining maxillary incisors; replacing maxillary canines and lateral incisors; restitution of anterior dental esthetics; vicissitudes of maxillary incisors
median maxillary diastema 110, 112, 115–116, 120, 121
metal-ceramic prostheses 60, 124

N

nightguard 25
NobelReplace fixture 77
non-malfeasance 5

O

oral hygiene 25
orthodontic treatment
    advantages 58
    disadvantages 58
orthognathic surgery
    advantages 58
    disadvantages 58

P

palatal bevel reduction 28, 29, 30
palatal chamfer reduction 28, 29, 30
palatal peninsular flap 45, 48
partial dentures *see* fixed partial dentures;
    removable partial dentures
patient needs and wants 6–7
PLVs *see* porcelain laminate veneers
polymerization shrinkage 33
porcelain laminate veneers (PLVs)
    advantages 12, 25
    bilayer 37
    CLVs vs 25
    disadvantages 12, 25
    as novel modality 91
    replacement treatment 64–68
    treatment sequences using 16–19, 26–35, 99–105
Procera laminate 37
prostheses, materials 60, 124

Index

R

recession 49
referral 6
removable partial dentures
    advantages 58, 72, 115
    disadvantages 44, 58, 72, 115
    transitional 74–75, 110, 112
replacing maxillary canines and lateral incisors 9–20
    clinical erudition and feasibility 12
    dental history 10
    discussion 20
    patient needs and wants 12–13
    postoperative status 9, 18–19
    preoperative status 9–10, 18–19
    scientific credence for treatment 12
    treatment options 10–11
    treatment sequence 13–19
resin-composite fillings *see* composite fillings
restitution of anterior dental esthetics 95–107
    clinical erudition and feasibility 97
    dental history 96
    discussion 106
    patient needs and wants 97
    postoperative status 95, 102–105, 107
    preoperative status 95, 96, 97, 102–106
    scientific credence for treatment 96–97
    treatment options 96
    treatment sequence 99–105
restorations
    guidelines 98
    margin locations 98, 100, 101
restorations
    material choice 98, 99–100
    types 98, 99
    see also restitution of anterior dental esthetics
restoring structural integrity and esthetics following tooth wear
    clinical erudition and feasibility 25
    dental history 22, 23
    discussion 37
    patient needs and wants 25
    postoperative status 21, 34–36
    preoperative status 21, 22, 23–24, 34–35
    scientific credence for treatment 22
    treatment options 22
    treatment sequence 26–35
Rochette bridges 56, 57, 114, 115
    advantages 115
    disadvantages 115
root fillings 64–65
root resorption 42

S

scarring 51, 124
scientific credence 3–4
silica ceramics 60, 99, 124
single maxillary central incisor with hopeless prognosis 109–124
    clinical erudition and feasibility 115
    dental history 110–112
    discussion 122–124
    patient needs and wants 115
single maxillary central incisor with hopeless prognosis
    postoperative status 109, 118, 120–123
    preoperative status 109, 112–113, 118, 122–123
    scientific credence for treatment 115
    treatment options 114
    treatment sequence 115–122
skill 5–6
subjectivity 2, 8, 93
survival rates 4, 5

T

titanium abutments 17, 79–81, 84, 118
tooth wear 22
    treatment methods 22
    see also restoring structural integrity and esthetics following tooth wear
traumatic loss of maxillary central incisors 55–62
    clinical erudition and feasibility 58
    dental history 56
    discussion 62
    patient needs and wants 58–60
    postoperative status 55, 62
    preoperative status 55–57, 61–62
    scientific credence for treatment 58, 59
    treatment options 58
    treatment sequence 60–61

Index

V

vicissitudes of maxillary incisors 63–93
   clinical crudition and feasibility 74
   dental history 64–71
   discussion 91–93
   patient needs and wants 74
   postoperative status 63, 90–92

vicissitudes of maxillary incisors 63–93
   preoperative status 63, 72
   scientific credence for treatment 72
   treatment options 72–73
   treatment sequence 74–91
      first try-in 84–87
      second try-in 87–88
      third try-in 88–89
      fourth try-in 89–90

W

window reduction 28–29, 30

Z

zirconia abutments 20, 48–50, 53, 82–84, 90, 118–121
zirconia ceramics 60, 100, 124